Gastrointestinal Symptoms

Gastrointestinal Symptoms

CLINICAL INTERPRETATION

J. Edward Berk, M.D., D.Sc.
Distinguished Professor of Medicine
University of California, Irvine

William S. Haubrich, M.D.
Clinical Professor of Medicine
University of California, San Diego
Senior Consultant Emeritus, Division of Gastroenterology
The Scripps Clinic and Research Foundation
La Jolla, California

B.C. Decker, Inc.
Philadelphia

Publisher	B.C. Decker Inc.
	320 Walnut Street
	Suite 400
	Philadelphia, Pennsylvania 19106

Sales and Distribution

United States and Puerto Rico
Mosby-Year Book Inc.
11830 Westline Industrial Drive
Saint Louis, Missouri 63146

Canada
Mosby-Year Book Limited
5240 Finch Ave. E., Unit 1
Scarborough, Ontario M1S 5A2

Australia
**McGraw-Hill Book Company
Australia Pty. Ltd.**
4 Barcoo Street
Roseville East 2069
New South Wales, Australia

Brazil
**Editora McGraw-Hill do Brasil,
Ltda.**
rua Tabapua, 1.105, Itaim-Bibi
Sao Paulo, S.P. Brasil

Colombia
**Interamericana/McGraw-Hill de
Colombia, S.A.**
Carrera 17, No. 33-71
(Apartado Postal, A.A., 6131)
Bogota, D.E., Colombia

*Europe, United Kingdom, Middle
East and Africa*
Wolfe Publishing Limited
Brook House
2-16 Torrington Place
London WC1E 7LT
England

Hong Kong and China
McGraw-Hill Book Company
Suite 618, Ocean Centre
5 Canton Road
Tsimshatsui, Kowloon
Hong Kong

India
**Tata McGraw-Hill Publishing
Company, Ltd.**
12/4 Asaf Ali Road, 3rd Floor
New Delhi 110002, India

Indonesia
Mr. Wong Fin Fah
P.O. Box 122/JAT
Jakarta, 1300 Indonesia

Japan
Igaku-Shoin Ltd.
Tokyo International P.O. Box 5063
1-28-36 Hongo, Bunkyo-ku,
Tokyo 113, Japan

Korea
Mr. Don-Gap Choi
C.P.O. Box 10583
Seoul, Korea

Malaysia
Mr. Lim Tao Slong
No. 8 Jalan SS 7/6B
Kelana Jaya
47301 Petaling Jaya
Selangor, Malaysia

Mexico
**Interamericana/McGraw-Hill de
Mexico, S.A. de C.V.**
Cedro 512, Colonia Atlampa
(Apartado Postal 26370)
06450 Mexico, D.F., Mexico

New Zealand
**McGraw-Hill Book Co. New
Zealand Ltd.**
5 Joval Place, Wiri
Manukau City, New Zealand

Portugal
**Editora McGraw-Hill de Portugal,
Ltda.**
Rua Rosa Damasceno 11A-B
1900 Lisboa, Portugal

Singapore and Southeast Asia
McGraw-Hill Book Co.
21 Neythal Road
Jurong, Singapore 2262

South Africa
Libriger Book Distributors
Warehouse Number 8
"Die Ou Looiery"
Tannery Road
Hamilton, Bloemfontein 9300

Spain
**McGraw-Hill/Interamericana de
Espana, S.A.**
Manuel Ferrero, 13
28020 Madrid, Spain

Taiwan
Mr. George Lim
P.O. Box 87-601
Taipei, Taiwan

Thailand
Mr. Vitit Lim
632/5 Phaholyothin Road
Sapan Kwai
Bangkok 10400
Thailand

Venezuela
**Editorial Interamericana de
Venezuela, C.A.**
2da. calle Bello Monte
Local G-2
Caracas, Venezuela

NOTICE

The authors and publisher have made every effort to ensure that the patient care recommended herein, including choice of drugs and drug dosages, is in accord with the accepted standards and practice at the time of publication. However, since research and regulation constantly change clinical standards, the reader is urged to check the product information sheet included in the package of each drug, which includes recommended doses, warnings, and contraindications. This is particularly important with new or infrequently used drugs.

Gastrointestinal Symptoms: Clinical Interpretation   ISBN 1-55664-196-6

Library of Congress catalog card number: 90-83568   10 9 8 7 6 5 4 3 2 1

To our teachers, colleagues, and students
—and especially to our patients—
who taught us to appreciate the value of the matters
that are the concern of this book.

CONTRIBUTORS

J. Edward Berk, M.D., D.Sc.
Distinguished Professor of Medicine,
    University of California, Irvine
    Diarrhea
Gaseousness
Anorexia

Barton J. Blinder, M.D., Ph.D.
Clinical Professor and Director, Eating
    Disorders Programs and Research
    Department of Psychiatry and
    Human Behavior, University of
    California, Irvine
Eating Disorders

Abraham Bogoch, M.D.,
    B.Sc.(Med.), D.Sc.
Emeritus Clinical Professor of
    Medicine, University of British
    Columbia Faculty of Medicine; Active
    Staff, Department of Medicine,
    Vancouver General Hospital, and
    Honorary Staff, University Hospital,
    Shaughnessy Site, Vancouver, British
    Columbia, Canada
Gastrointestinal Bleeding

William S. Haubrich, M.D.
Clinical Professor of Medicine,
    University of California, San Diego;
    Senior Consultant Emeritus,
    Division of Gastroenterology,
    Scripps Clinic & Research
    Foundation, La Jolla, California
Abdominal Pain
Nausea and Vomiting
Weight Loss
Diarrhea
Disturbed Oral and Nasal Sensations

John C. Hoefs, M.D.
Associate Professor of Medicine and
    Director, Liver Disease Program,
    University of California, Irvine
Ascites

Walter J. Hogan, M.D.
Professor of Medicine, Medical College
    of Wisconsin, Milwaukee, Wisconsin
Heartburn
Swallowing Problems: Dysphagia and
    Odynophagia

G. *Gordon McHardy, M.D.*
Emeritus Professor of Medicine,
  Louisiana State University School of
  Medicine, New Orleans, Louisiana
Diarrhea

Arvey I. Rogers, M.D.
Professor of Medicine, University of
  Miami School of Medicine; Chief,
  Gastroenterology Section, Veterans
  Administration Medical Center,
  Miami, Florida
Constipation

Henry J. Tumen, M.D.
Emeritus Professor of Medicine,
  University of Pennsylvania School
  of Medicine; Director of Medical
  Education, Graduate Hospital,
  Philadelphia, Pennsylvania
Jaundice

Stewart G. Wolf, M.D.
Professor of Medicine, Temple
  University School of Medicine,
  Philadelphia; Director, Totts Gap
  Medical Research Laboratory,
  Bangor, Pennsylvania
History Taking: The Art of Dialogue

PREFACE

"Listen to the patient—he will tell you the diagnosis." Wise indeed was this admonition of a medical sage of yesteryear.

Patients consult a physician because of symptoms that are distressing or worrisome. Still to be devised is a machine capable of competing with a perceptive and astute physician in eliciting, understanding, and interpreting these symptoms. Yet, detailed solicitation and precise description of what actually troubles the patient seem all too often to be given short shrift. Insufficiently appreciated as well is the fine distinction between a "symptom" and a "complaint." Witness, for example, the woman who uncomplainingly endures heartburn for years, even neglecting to mention it (unless or until specifically asked) when driven to consult her doctor because of difficulty swallowing. She has had a "symptom" (heartburn) but for her it is not a "complaint." Consider similarly the man who placidly pursues his daily chores despite a liver riddled with cancer from a previously resected cancer of the colon. He clearly has "disease," but is not "ill" and is not complaining. In contrast is his neighbor, a woman with an irritable bowel who tells all who will listen (including, on innumerable visits, her doctor) of her torment. The neighbor has an abundance of symptoms, all uttered as complaints, and considers herself ill, as indeed she is in the sense that there is disturbed function of a bodily structure. Although she is in no real jeopardy, her subjective response to the derangement renders her pitifully distraught. These simple examples illustrate that, as physicians, we have a good deal to sort out in evaluating our patients.

All of us who undertake to solve clinical problems, perhaps especially those involving the digestive system, have come to rely heavily on the laboratory, imaging methods, endoscopy, and other special techniques that aid us in establishing our diagnoses. We are grateful, of course, for the advances in technology that have engendered these resources and enhanced our diagnostic prowess. There are times and circumstances, however, wherein we may become unduly reliant on such tools to furnish a diagnosis. It is all too easy to succumb to the fallacy of "5 minutes of history and 5 days of tests." A purposeful effort to elicit a thorough history often can guide us to a more discriminating choice of tests or narrow the need to fewer tests. Attentiveness to the patient's complaints, and ferreting out unproferred associated symptoms, fortified by a careful, informed, and perceptive analysis of the information so obtained may well, in the long run, save time, conserve valuable resources, reduce risk, and lessen the cost of diagnosis.

Concern about these matters, and a desire to reawaken interest in them, motivated the preparation of this book. The primary aim is to reaffirm the fundamental role of clinical symptom evaluation in the diagnosis of gastrointestinal disorders. To this end, the component chapters center on the thought processes that the clinician follows in seeking to elucidate and assess the complaints presented by a given patient. Concentration is on clinical diagnostic evaluation, based on the history and physical findings within the setting of the office, the clinic, or the bedside.

Initiated by a discourse on history taking and the art of dialogue, the chapters that follow deal with the principal symptoms or physical changes that relate to the digestive system. The nature of these symptoms, or such alterations as jaundice and ascites, makes rigid uniformity in presentation neither possible nor desirable. In each chapter, however, the underlying mechanisms, the clinical features, and key clinical pointers that may help in eliciting and interpreting a given symptom are stressed. Brief mention is also made of more objective studies that may confirm or exclude the impressions formed from clinical analysis alone. Wherever suitable, illustrative cases are narrated to highlight and underscore important elements.

The contributors of the component essays are all seasoned gastroenterologic clinicians who share in common a deep appreciation of symptom evaluation in the diagnostic process. If their expositions should succeed in directing attention to the need to probe, analyze, and interpret symptoms arising from digestive disturbances, the purpose of this work will have been most gratifyingly met.

To our colleagues who so kindly contributed to this work, we extend our thanks for their willingness to share their knowledge and experience. We are grateful to them as well for their gracious responses to the many requests we made of them.

We also wish to acknowledge our indebtedness and express our gratitude to Ms. Mary Mansor, Medical Editor, B.C. Decker, Inc., for her unfailing encouragement and sage advice.

J. Edward Berk, M.D., D.Sc.
William S. Haubrich, M.D.

CONTENTS

HISTORY TAKING:
THE ART OF DIALOGUE

Stewart G. Wolf, M.D.

1

History taking, the initial step in the patient–physician encounter, perhaps more than any other aspect of the diagnostic process, differentiates the highly skilled physician from his or her more plodding and less perceptive colleague. History taking is a high art that must be carried out in such a way as to enable the patient to respond to questions in a frank and unguarded manner. He or she must be made to feel safe and reassured that, no matter what is said in the doctor's presence, there is no danger of censure, ridicule, or betrayal. Through the dialogue, the physician's ears and eyes must be alert to subtle and fleeting cues that may illuminate the patient's account of the illness and thereby lead to relevant directions of diagnostic inquiry and to helpful tactics in therapy.

I have often asked consultants what enabled them to arrive at a correct diagnosis that had eluded the referring physician. Nearly always, the crucial clue had come from something the patient had said or the way in which he or she had said it.

Today, gastroenterologists can make a positive tissue diagnosis in a very large proportion of digestive system lesions through endoscopy or biopsy. The decision to carry out these invasive and uncomfortable procedures, however, should be guided by the findings of a thorough and penetrating history. Moreover, the history may add etiologic evidence to an otherwise purely anatomic finding. Also, as it facilitates understanding of the patient, the history may provide valuable leads to effective treatment and recruitment of the patient as a cooperating partner in the therapeutic plan.

Establishing Rapport

Skill in gaining a patient's confidence is not merely a matter of technique. It depends on the physician's personal qualifications, interest and belief in people, and ability to give encouragement and support even in the face of the patient's intransigence or hostility.

Success or failure in communication often depends heavily on the patient's initial impression of the physician. Repeatedly, one hears patients say of a physician, "He's such a busy man that I didn't want to burden him with my troubles" or "He didn't have time to talk to me." The physician who, even unintentionally, has given the patient such an impression has placed himself or herself at a disadvantage and has perhaps denied himself or herself important diagnostic data.

"History taking is best done in private, without interruption, and by the physician."

Other reactions to an encounter with a physician were "I was a little afraid of him" or "He didn't seem interested" or "He seemed to be having troubles of his own." These remarks imply, of course, a defect in the attitude of the physician who was unable to put the patient at ease and inspire his or her confidence. Confidence and trust are fostered when history taking is done in private, without interruption, and by the physician himself or herself. Furthermore, subtle and valuable clues to the diagnosis often emerge in the initial encounter. Perceptions and intuitions honed and refined by training and experience can be processed by no computer other than the human one—the physician's brain.

The history is a useful device for getting to know and understand the patient, but its main purpose is to evaluate evidence that may lead to a correct diagnosis and may help to guide therapy. The history is not an exercise in serial questions and answers; on the contrary, it is an instrument that can be effectively applied only in proportion to the skill of the physician. Simply asking all the prescribed questions will not necessarily provide useful clues to the patient's problem. The history should take the form of an inquiry in which one piece of information leads to another. Although the process of history taking must be thorough, there is no such thing as a complete history. Each history differs from every other, depending on the nature of the patient and his or her illness. The history remains the most powerful diagnostic tool because diagnosis is still in essence an intellectual process, an exercise in clinical analysis. Technical aids can be of enormous help but cannot replace the physician's perspicacity and reasoning power. To supplement effectively his or her radiologic and electronic diagnostic tools, as well as his or her endoscopes and imaging techniques, the physician must know how to elicit as well as to evaluate pertinent historical data.

Medical curricula once required students to refine the diagnostic possibilities by a penetrating analysis of the clinical data, allowing only a parsimonious approach to laboratory testing. Today, however, it is common practice to order occasionally irrelevant, often costly, and sometimes arduous and uncomfortable diagnostic procedures on the outside chance that "something might be picked up." The very multiplicity of tests in such a diagnostic strategy increases the opportunity for error and the risk of accident. Appropriate sophisticated tests and procedures many times are indispensable in confirming a correct diagnosis; however, just as often they are not needed at all. Premature testing without adequate attention to the data directly available from the history and physical examination is always wasteful and may actually derail the diagnostic inquiry.

The following case illustrates the baneful consequences of substituting tests and referrals for the traditional dialogue with the patient.

☐ *Illustrative Case*

Mr. Taylor was 56 years old when he became concerned about discomfort in his upper abdomen, mainly on the right side. He was not sure how long he had felt it, but it seemed to have been getting more troublesome recently. "It was not exactly a pain," he said, "more of an aching or a sense of fullness." Occasionally he would be nauseated after meals. Nothing of significance was elicited by review of his previous medical history except for periodic episodes of urticaria over the past several years. Mr. Taylor worked in an editorial office of a newspaper, had not traveled outside of the United States, and had no known contact with tuberculosis, toxic chemicals, or other suspicious environmental agents.

"Studies made without attention to the data obtained from the history and physical findings may derail diagnosis."

Physical examination disclosed slight icterus, a fever of 100°F, slight tenderness in the right upper quadrant, and an indefinite right upper quadrant mass that was thought to be either liver or gallbladder.

The attending physician ordered a urinalysis, a complete blood count, liver function tests, and a radiographic examination of the gallbladder. The urine revealed no abnormalities, and the blood count was unremarkable except for a slight eosinophilia. The gallbladder radiograph was normal. The tests of hepatic function showed only a moderate elevation of bilirubin, mainly in the direct fraction.

On the strength of these findings, and the persistence of low-grade fever, the physician abandoned his initial impression of gallbladder disease and began to suspect cancer, either primary in the liver or metastatic from some other site. A liver scintiscan was ordered, and it showed a solitary nodule approximately 3 cm in diameter that did not take up the radioactive contrast medium.

At this point, the physician admitted Mr. Taylor to the hospital for a battery of tests and radiographs in search of a primary source for a metastasis in the liver; none was found. The fever, slight icterus, and tenderness in the right upper quadrant persisted. After 2 weeks in the hospital—at a cost of nearly $14,000 for room and board, nursing care, tests, radiographs, and consultations—a needle biopsy of the liver was attempted; however, the nodule apparently was located too deep for the needle to reach.

One Sunday morning, as the puzzled but determined physician was making his rounds and seriously considering exploratory surgery, he noted that his patient was reading a foreign newspaper with printing in another language. "It's Greek," explained the patient. "It's the paper we publish here for Greek-speaking people." "But your name—are you Greek?" asked the physician. The patient explained that he had come to the United States at 12 years of age with his parents, and that the immigration clerk had recorded his father's name as an anglicized version of the name his father had pronounced in Greek.

This small item of information, which would have turned up in a proper medical history, immediately suggested the correct diagnosis: an echinococcus cyst. This disorder is commonly encountered in Mediterranean countries, including Greece, but is seen rarely in the United States, and then usually in patients who were infected earlier elsewhere. It is well known that an echinococcus cyst may form and remain in the liver for many years without producing symptoms.

Comment.   Had the Greek connection been brought out initially and linked to the history of urticaria and the slight eosinophilia, the patient would have been spared 2 weeks of hospital confinement and discomfort. Furthermore, the financial cost of the diagnosis and treatment would have been much reduced.

Technical Considerations

"It is much more important that pertinent information be recorded in the doctor's mind than on a card or in a file." Lack of thoroughness in establishing the patient's background, evident in the case of the patient just cited, is only one among many pitfalls that may seriously hinder a diagnostic inquiry. Another is faulty reasoning, relying on the volume instead of the pertinence of the data;

believing, like Conan Doyle's Inspector Lestrade, that toting up the clues will lead to a correct diagnosis. In contrast, the skilled diagnostician keeps his or her intellectual motor running during history taking. Instead of simply compiling the data and judging it later, he or she begins to consider likely diagnoses from the moment of first greeting the patient, or shortly thereafter. Then, like Sherlock Holmes,* the physician may approach a correct diagnosis by pursuing a bit of evidence that does not fit an otherwise plausible impression. At this point, the selection of appropriate confirmatory tests or procedures can be made with maximal economy and precision.

Physicians who practice medicine with such an attitude of active inquiry, exercising keen senses and incisive reasoning, usually enjoy the greatest prestige among their medical colleagues. Today, unfortunately, diminishing numbers of physicians are willing to take on such an elaborate, painstaking, but satisfying intellectual exercise. Some leave the history taking to a relatively untutored assistant or to a computer terminal. Others may have the physical examinations of their patients performed by a surrogate. The resulting body of data, collected by less practiced eyes and ears and without the sensitive nose of a trained medical sleuth, will likely suggest two or three, or even more, diagnostic possibilities. Some of these would have been eliminated promptly by careful attention to incompatible data.

Teaching the Art of Interviewing

With the aim of sharpening students' perceptions of important clues and encouraging continuous attention to potentially significant data, my associates and I monitored and recorded history taking by fourth-year medical students in the outpatient clinic. Verbatim quotes from the recordings led to quick recognition of weaknesses in a student's method of interviewing, which could be classified as errors of commission or omission.

Errors of Commission

- By seeking rapid accurate answers to a prepared list of questions and failing to frame their questions in view of replies to earlier ones, students lost the opportunity to make of the history an exploration whose direction is suggested by each previous step. Moreover, they failed to take into account the possibility that many questions may elicit answers that may be politely or protectively misleading or entirely incorrect.
- By forcing the patient to express his or her "chief complaint" in a few words, students often failed to get on the right track. Sometimes the chief

---

* It is more than coincidence that Sir Arthur Conan Doyle patterned the perspicacity of the famous detective after that of his former medical preceptor, the astute diagnostician Dr. Joseph Bell of Edinburgh.

complaint as recorded by the student contained a plausible excuse for the visit but did not reflect the patient's real reasons for seeking help. Since the handling of subsequent portions of the history is inevitably influenced by the content of the chief complaint, inadequacy at this stage may lead to a misdirected and largely irrelevant inquiry.

- Students often did too much of the talking themselves, phrasing questions in such a manner that they could be answered "yes" or "no." Such an approach not only deprives the examiner of the shades of meaning that a patient can communicate by a less direct answer, but also denies the examiner important leads frequently inherent in a patient's relatively informal description of his or her difficulties.

- Often, the converse of the error described above was made by the same student, at another time in the interview, by allowing the patient to engage in a long, circumstantial account of details of symptoms and thus failing to bring the problem into focus. Occasionally, the interview assumed the tone of a social conversation, with the student interrupting the patient now and then to utter words of sympathy or approbation while failing to gather useful data.

"Questions may be worded so as to elicit misleading or incorrect answers."

- At times, lack of taste and discretion was evident on the part of the student in phrasing questions and in attempting to deal with the patient's natural reticence in discussing personal matters. An off-hand approach or an introductory remark such as "Now I am going to ask about your personal life" often put the patient on guard unnecessarily, so that later questions yielded only euphemisms or actual misinformation. The sensibilities of some patients were offended by such questions as "How's the sex life?" or "Did you ever have gonorrhea or syphilis?" Some of the students' questions were phrased in a fashion entirely unsuited to the patient; for example, a candidate for a doctorate in a scientific field was questioned about "making water" rather than about "urinating." A 14-year-old, slow-witted schoolboy was asked "Do you repress resentment?"

Errors of Omission

- Important leads were many times provided by the patient's spontaneous remarks, the wording used in reply, or an accompanying gesture, but the students frequently failed to follow up on these clues. An event or circumstance might be noted, and even recorded, by the student, without being considered in the formulation of the diagnosis. Similarly, a student might fail to ascertain and weigh the results of diagnostic and therapeutic procedures.

- Difficulties arose because of insufficient awareness of the individual peculiarities among patients or of a particular patient's limitations in communicating, so that the patient's observations were too easily accepted at face value. For example, a patient's statement that she had never had tarry stools was not doubted until inquiry by the instructor revealed that the patient never looked at her stools. Similarly, reports of a "cold" or "heart attack" were sometimes accepted without asking for supporting evidence.

- Often, because of preoccupation with charting procedures, valuable leads that could be gained from observing the tone and quality of the patient's voice, slips of the tongue, misinterpretations, or contradictory statements were lost. Some students also ignored fairly obvious signs such as facial expressions in response to certain questions, flushing, tears, sweating, or changes in respiration.

Defects in the technique of communication such as these are common in the inexperienced clinician. Without sufficient training and practice, they may form the basis of habits that hamper effective history taking throughout a physician's practicing career.

"Defects in communication technique may become habitual and hamper effective history taking."

Contribution of the History to Diagnostic Precision

The gastroenterologist's diagnostic precision can be abetted considerably by sensitivity to subtle cues in a patient's statements and behavior because, as it is widely acknowledged, 80 percent or more of complaints presented to the physician reflect disturbances in gastrointestinal function. Gastrointestinal function, in turn, is regulated by an interactive neurohumoral network under the strong influence of forebrain structures that interpret and formulate responses to life experience. My colleagues and I, as well as others, have shown that influences from these higher centers may powerfully affect, either consciously or unconsciously, salivary, esophageal, gastric, biliary, pancreatic, intestinal, colonic, and rectal mechanisms. Recently, it has been discovered that these influences are capable of altering not only hormonal but also immune processes.

The important central neural circuits served by the peripheral autonomic pathways leading to smooth muscles, glands, and secretory cells may set in motion a whole gamut of symptomatic and potentially harmful gastrointestinal disturbances. These disturbances and the symptoms associated with them may respond more or less to a wide array of medications; however, to understand the etiology of the disturbance often requires understanding of the patient.

The following excerpt illustrates how one patient's alarming gastrointestinal symptoms—which could not have been explained by any amount of costly endoscopy, electronic recordings, or imaging—were illuminated by, and ultimately yielded to, a skillfully conducted interview.

Illustrative Case

For 8 weeks, Mr. C., 24 years old, had been experiencing anorexia, nausea, and vomiting so severe that he had lost more than 20 pounds. After the patient's family history and personal medical history had been noted, the student turned to the present illness and learned that the patient's symptoms had begun on the day of his marriage. Further questioning elicited another concurrent problem: premature ejaculation. The student jumped to the conclusion that there was a disturbance in the patient's psychosexual development—perhaps ambivalence about his role as a man or perhaps a homosexual tendency. Accordingly, he carefully reviewed the patient's early sexual experience, inquired extensively about his first meeting with his wife, their courtship, and their wedding night. The patient answered all questions in an earnest and frank manner, obviously eager to cooperate, but nothing pertinent was revealed. Fortunately, the interview had been recorded, and on replay the student picked up the clue that he had missed while taking the family history. A portion of the exchange follows:

Student: You're married?
Patient: Yes, I was married June twenty-fourth, this year.
Student: Is your wife from Omaha?
Patient: No, she's from Fort Madison, but we were married in Omaha, hoping my mother would come. She only gets around in a wheelchair.
Student: Yes, you mentioned that your mother had had an accident. You have no children, then?

While listening to the recording, the student realized that he had missed the significant lead: "hoping my mother would come."

At the next visit, the pertinent part of the story quickly unfolded. The patient's mother had been rendered paraplegic in an automobile accident that occurred while he was driving. He had been seriously injured also but had recovered. His mother apparently had adjusted to her disability remarkably well and gave no indication of resentment toward him. His father had died 2 years earlier. An older brother and two older sisters were married, so the patient continued to live at home. His mother ran the household, and a nurse and a maid looked after her personal needs.

The patient's mother had never shown any particular enthusiasm about any of the women in whom he was interested, but she had been pleasant and cordial whenever he brought one of them to the house. When the patient finally became engaged, his mother seemed to accept the prospect of marriage but gave no special encouragement. He was uneasy and felt guilty about leaving her.

His mother's failure to appear at the wedding, which had been especially arranged by the bride's parents to be conveniently accessible to his mother, was a severe blow to the patient. He managed to repress his feelings, however, until the facts were elicited during the second interview. Then, as the realization struck him, the patient wept a bit and talked a great deal. The student listened and reassured the patient that his mother was naturally frightened of, and perhaps angry at, losing him, but that she would probably accept this event with the same equanimity with which she had accepted other difficult situations. Following that interview, the patient's symptoms improved rapidly, and by the next visit a week later they had subsided entirely.

Comment.   Had the interview not been recorded, the student's initial error—missing the important clue in the family history—probably would have steered the student away from the correct diagnosis and toward a series of unnecessary tests and radiographs.

Counterproductive Techniques for Data Gathering

Illustrative Case

The approach of another student, who suspected that marital conflict contributed to his patient's gastrointestinal symptoms, could be described as "inquisitional." His rapid-fire questions fell like blows from a triphammer, threatening his patient's sense of privacy. Moreover, instead of waiting for replies, he suggested answers to his patient, a 53-year-old housewife who complained of epigastric distress.

Student: How old were you when you got married?
Patient: Forty.
Student: You were 40 when you got married. Had you had many opportunities to get married before that? Just waiting for the right man, or . . . what was it?
Patient: I didn't care.
Student: You didn't care. I don't understand . . . you didn't care. You mean you had no desire to get—
Patient: I had opportunities . . .
Student: But?
Patient: But I was making plenty of money at that time . . .
Student: And to make the money was more important than to get married and start a family?

Patient: I was always afraid I wouldn't get the right man.
Student: You were? Why?
Patient: I don't know.
Student: What was the matter? Had you had some bad experiences in your own family?
Patient: No. I saw a few other people, friends of mine . . .
Student: Yes.
Patient: So I figured, "take it easy—plenty of time."
Student: Did you have a lot of boyfriends?
Patient: Yes.
Student: How old was your husband? Was he older than you or younger?
Patient: He was in his forties.
Student: In his late forties? How much older was your husband than you?
Patient: Five years older.
Student: Five? Where did you meet him?
Patient: Do I have to tell you all that?
Student: No, you don't have to. It is perfectly all right. I don't care.

Comment.   This student's final statement reflected more clearly than he realized his attitude toward his patient. A physician who doesn't care will rarely be able to communicate effectively with sick people.

*"**A** physician who doesn't care will rarely be able to communicate effectively."*

Illustrative Case

Occasionally, indifference to and obliviousness of the patient as a person is reflected in a thoughtless, overstructured routine of questioning that almost precludes useful information. A student's dialogue with a Mrs. F., an extremely tense 48-year-old white married woman who complained of frequent loose stools, illustrates not only indifference and gaucherie, as did the previous case, but also cursoriness and lack of curiosity.

Patient: I just got married; it must be about four and a half years ago.
Student: Had you ever considered marriage before that?
Patient: Oh yes, a couple of times before that.
Student: How often do you take some kind of whiskey or beer?
Patient: I haven't had a drink in over a year. I don't smoke either, except once in a while to be sociable, but I haven't even done that since I've been sick.
Student: How much sleep do you get at night?
Patient: Well . . . I try to get about eight hours every night, but I don't get that.

At this point it was apparent to the instructor that this patient had always had a shaky relationship with the opposite sex and that facts about her relationship with her husband might be pertinent to her colitis. Since the student was getting nowhere with his pursuit of the evidence, the instructor interrupted the dialogue. Feeling the need to preserve continuity in the questioning so that the patient would not feel threatened by a sudden change of topic, the instructor, in a quiet and gentle voice, took over the interview.

Instructor: Has your husband been drinking at all?

Patient: He doesn't drink either, or smoke. [A long pause ensues here during which the patient seems to be preparing some further statement about her husband (Fig. 1–1).] My husband is at least ten years older than me, and that may explain some of our differences. I say, at least ten years older, because, when we first met, he told me that he was ten years older; but since, I have reason to believe that he is more than ten years older than I am. I don't know whether that means anything, except that we don't think alike on many things . . . and he clings to very, very old-fashioned ideas about almost everything, and he has something to say about everything, including things that I don't think concern him . . . like things about the house, furniture, curtains, or anything. He will come in the kitchen . . . you know, something I am cooking . . . well, he thinks he knows more about cooking than I do. He has something to say about everything.

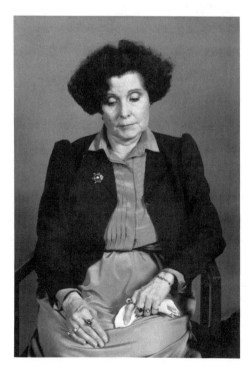

FIGURE 1–1. Mrs. M., during a long pause in her reply to a question about her husband, appears pensive but awkward, with downcast eyes suggesting ambivalent feelings about him. (This is a simulation of the actual posture and expression of the patient.) (Courtesy of Jane Chew Deckert, M.S.)

Instructor: How much do you think these things have to do with your health?

Patient: Well, I think that must have quite a bit to do with it. I hate to say it [begins to cry at this point] but in my heart I feel . . . that . . . I don't like . . . I don't like to break up my marriage . . . but I realize that . . . my husband was not the person . . . I should have married. It was only about six months after we were married that he struck me . . . just in a fit of temper over some silly little thing that didn't concern him.

Comment.   Often by carefully watching the patient, it is possible to know that a single question is all that may be needed to bring out relevant material. However, preoccupation with charting and being in a hurry to get to the next question may interfere with opportunities for such observations.

> "**B**y carefully watching the patient, it may be possible to select the question or questions needed to bring out relevant material."

A Productive Approach to Data Gathering

Illustrative Case

One student who gave free rein to the patient to develop his own story collected considerable pertinent data in a relatively short time. His patient, Mr. G., a 30-year-old salesman, had a chronic complaint of anorexia and nausea.

Student: Tell me a little bit about what brings you here.

Patient: Actually, it's my stomach. I've been suffering with my stomach on and off since I was in the army. During the past five years I went to the doctor. Once, a couple of years back, I had a check-up, went on a diet, and was told to gain some weight, but I never did. I suffer indigestion quite a bit, don't gain weight, feel tired and rundown, so I thought I'd better come down and see if there was anything wrong.

Student: You've been to a number of doctors in the past five years?

Patient: I have. I went to my own family doctor and he recommended that I go to a specialist for some x-rays. So I went through a set of x-rays and they didn't find anything at that time, but that was about three years ago.

Student: The last time you were well was five years ago?

Patient: I think it was even more than that, because all the time I was in the army I never ate right; when all the other guys were gaining weight and eating like horses, I never ate. I never could eat breakfast and I never felt right.

Student: Can you tell me then the last time you were well, as far as your stomach is concerned?

Patient: I think it was back twenty years ago. Well, even as a youngster I had a weak stomach . . . I mean, it was easily upset. I'd get faint very easily; if I went for a needle or a shot or a Wassermann, I'd get faint and things would upset my stomach. I'd get that sick, nauseous feeling very easily, you know. Now that I think back, I always had a weak stomach.

Comment.   During this brief preliminary history, the patient was allowed to speak without any pressure from the student, to whom it quickly became apparent that he was dealing with a life-long pattern of gastrointestinal symptoms. He also noted the patient's childish mannerisms of speech and tone and voice, which prompted him to investigate the patient's background and social adjustment for its possible bearing on his gastrointestinal disorder.

Illustrative Case

In contrast, the approach of another student to his patient, Miss G., illustrates the self-defeating effect of awkward attempts at precision, hoping to get "just the facts, ma'am."

Patient: I left the house feeling perfectly all right; I live in Queens. I got on at Ninetieth Street Station, and before I reached Woodside on the local, I began to feel kind of peculiar feelings in my stomach, no actual pain, but I might say nauseous . . .
Student: Where did you feel that?
Patient: In through here . . . and . . .
Student: And you felt sick at your stomach?
Patient: Yes. And I get off at Queens Plaza and go across the platform to the BMT, which takes me to Lexington Avenue; it goes down into the subway. Well, when I got down underground, the perspiration just poured off me as if I was under a shower . . .
Student: This was in the evening?
Patient: No, in the morning.
Student: In the morning. Were the subways crowded?
Patient: Oh, yes. I was standing up . . .
Student: And you had a sick feeling right there?
Patient: It started there, as I say, and it seemed when I got into the subway, underground, the perspiration just poured off me. I had this same suit on . . . and when it was all over . . . I felt that it had gone clear through the suit that I had on.
Student: You were coming back from what, then, shopping?
Patient: I was going to work.
Student: You were going to work. What kind of work do you do now?
Patient: I'm with the New York City Housing Authority . . .
Student: What kind of work?
Patient: Stenography and typing.
Student: Stenography and typing.
Patient: And . . . I ordinarily change at Lexington Avenue, and I got off there. I

was afraid I was going to faint, although I've never fainted in my life. Things started to get gray and black . . . I just hung on, to this bar . . .

Student: This wasn't pain?

Patient: Well, combined with . . . I think the perspiration, I believe, started after the pain in the . . .

Student: Yes, but was it the pain or was it an uncomfortable feeling?

Patient: It was a sharp pain, it was just a . . . well, I don't know . . . it was a kind of a . . .

Student: Dull?

Patient: . . . Digestive pain, that's what I think it . . .

Student: Yes, but did it feel dull, was it aching?

Patient: Yes, it was a dull pain, it wasn't a sharp pain.

Student: It was dull. Was it more discomfort or pain?

Patient: Discomfort.

Student: Yes. Did it move up into your chest or down into your lower abdomen?

Patient: No.

Comment. About the only objective accomplished by this staccato rhythm of questioning is the interruption of the patient's account of her symptoms, which might have turned out to be coherent and informative.

Questions must provoke informative answers. Inability to elicit useful personal data often is caused by the way questions are asked. "What kind of things were you punished for as a child?" is a much better question than "Did your parents punish you very much?" The answer to the latter is "No" automatically, because no one wishes to criticize their own parents. Since every child is punished for something, the bases for parental punishment provide information on values and illuminate the atmosphere in which the patient grew up. Questions that invite euphemistic or platitudinous replies, that gloss over the problem, must be avoided; questions should stimulate the patient to think about himself or herself.

> *"The history taker's questions should stimulate the patient to think about himself or herself."*

It is especially important to avoid superficial conventional replies like those that a greeting such as "Hello, how are you?" might elicit from a friend who had been celebrating too much the night before. Instead of stopping to say, "Well, I'll tell you. I've got this epigastric sensation here, which is uncomfortable, and a little headache," the friend would probably walk by saying, "Fine, thanks, how are you?" Patients make similar socially acceptable responses to unskillful questioning.

An approach commonly practiced by physicians is to ask a few direct questions, hoping to cover the most likely areas of conflict, but which elicit instead a "Fine, thanks, how are you?" reply. Examples include:

How are things at home?
Does your wife nag?
Do the children annoy you?
Have you and your wife made a good sexual adjustment?
Do you have financial worries?
How are things at the job?
Do you get on well with your fellow workers?
Are there any worries that you can think of?

Such questions may elicit the required information from a few patients who already have considerable awareness of their problems and are not too diffident to discuss them. However, most patients will give benign partial answers to these questions, leaving the physician at a loss to know what to say next. It is best to avoid such blind alleys and instead to ask questions that require descriptive rather than "Yes" or "No" answers. A better question than "Is your boss unreasonable?" is "Tell me about the people you work with."

The patient's choice of words and tone of voice, as well as subtle implications of gesture and behavior, may speak volumes. Personal conflict may be suggested by a patient's unaccountable memory lapse or failure to mention important people or events in his or her life.

> *"Useful information may be gleaned by getting the patient to talk freely."*

For example, the president of a women's dress factory, who had had one of his most severe attacks of migraine headache a few days before, told his physician that that day had been free of stress—indeed, totally uneventful. When asked to recount his every move from the time he arose in the morning, however, he remembered that the headache came on while he was driving to the airport to pick up his father-in-law, the chairman of the board of the company, who had flown up from Florida to question why the last quarter's earnings had slumped.

Useful information can be gleaned whenever a patient can be induced to talk freely. Experts in interrogating prisoners-of-war have learned that when a prisoner is encouraged to talk freely about any subject he or she chooses, the prisoner will likely betray considerable useful information, often without being aware of having done so. Similarly, patients reveal a good deal about themselves when they talk. Unlike the prisoner, however, what a patient reveals may ultimately redound to his benefit. Unfortunately, even an experienced physician may wittingly or unwittingly take charge of the interview, suggesting answers to the patient instead of, by sparing his or her own words, inviting the patient to talk.

History Taking by Experienced Physicians

Illustrative Case

The patient, Dr. F., was a 40-year-old dentist of Russian-Jewish parentage who suffered from peptic ulcer and migraine headaches. He was welcomed into the office by the physician, a careful and thorough practitioner who had been in practice for 16 years and, impressed with the importance of taking a careful history, had begun to record his interviews. After the patient had described in detail his symptoms and past illnesses, and following a physical examination that failed to turn up any abnormality, the physician resumed the interview—a bit uneasily—as follows.

Physician: As you probably know, a good many physicians connect ulcer and migraine with emotional problems, so I think it would be well if we reviewed the situation together a little bit. Of course, you realize that anything you say to me is entirely confidential.

Patient: Yes, I know that, doctor, and I've given this thing considerable thought myself. I thought there might be some nervousness or emotional troubles, but for the life of me I can't find a thing. I've got a fine wife, two lovely children, an excellent practice, and a house of my own. We have no in-law troubles, and I should be the happiest man in the world.

Physician: Well, tell me some of the details. Is there any disturbance at home? Do the children get on your nerves?

[This line and several others were pursued with negative results and finally the physician asked the following questions.]

Physician: Well, what about the office? Is there anything down at the office that isn't going well? The landlord, your secretary, the place itself? Are you making as much in practice as you had hoped to?

Patient: Really, doctor, I'm doing better than I ever expected. I can't complain of my practice in any respect. It's as good as that of any dentist I know.

This physician approached the problem in an earnest and systematic way but got nowhere for the following reasons:

- By separating and even highlighting the discussion of his patient's personality adjustment, he had put Dr. F. on the defensive. The data gained could have been elicited along with the rest of the history or even during the physical examination.
- The physician's questions suggested possible points of conflict without his really knowing anything about Dr. F., including his hopes, fears, and aspirations.

A second physician, to whom this patient was referred, was able to bring into focus one factor of significant personal conflict in an interview that lasted the same length of time as that of the first physician. An excerpt of the interview with the second physician follows.

Physician: Are you doing with your life what you wanted to do?

Patient: [Long pause.] I can't be definite about that, doctor. I believe I am. I think I'm content.

Physician: What kind of practice did you plan for yourself when you first started out?

Patient: Well, that might be a source of discontent to myself. I have a fairly busy practice and I don't think its . . . perhaps the quality isn't there. And that might be a source of discontent in my own mind.

Physician: You mean that it's too routine?

Patient: Well, I think perhaps seeing too many patients, and you can't be as selective in your work; your quality is perhaps not as good as you'd like it to be. Now, I might be theorizing there.

Physician: Well, go ahead.

Patient: Those are possibilities that loom in my mind. I—I . . . uh, I have a busy practice, but perhaps it isn't a happy practice, though, in my own mind . . .

Physician: What would you . . . suppose all stops were out—what would you like to be doing?

Patient: Just what you're doing now. I've often thought I'd like to be affiliated with a university. I know I enjoyed my residency and internship immensely. I stayed on for about five years and I got a big bang out of that. I was very happy there.

Physician: When was this?

Patient: After I graduated, then interned. I stayed on as a resident.

Physician: And then did you think at the time of continuing in full time work, teaching?

Patient: Well, I opened an office not far from the hospital so that I could retain my position at the institution.

Physician: You still do that?

Patient: No, I gave that up. I guess somehow or other I got into a—I just got into a routine; we get ourselves married and we get into that sort of swing, as it were.

Physician: The need for better income?

Patient: I would imagine so.

Here Dr. F.'s manner was grim and dejected, and it was evident that an important area of conflict had been discovered (Fig. 1–2). The discussion moved logically to the question of the financial demands and social ambitions of Dr. F.'s wife. Soon the story of feeling caught in a treadmill, trying to supply the demands of an avid and ambitious wife, came out in clear relief. Dr. F. wept during much of this discussion, but at the end he said that he felt much relieved in having been able to discuss matters that were so close to him that he was hardly aware of them.

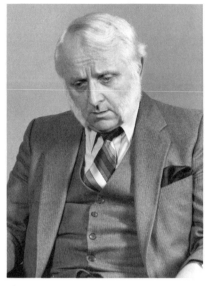
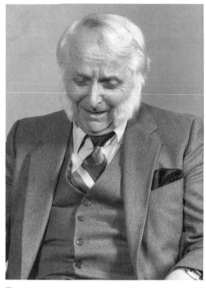

A   B

FIGURE 1-2. *A and B,* The patient, Dr. F., as he gradually becomes aware of his frustration and resentment at having had to sacrifice his academic aspirations to his wife's urge toward "upward mobility." (This is a simulation of the actual postures and expressions of the patient.) (Courtesy of Gordon H. Deckert, M.D.)

Comment.   It is important to note that Dr. F. was trying to be honest with both physicians. He had truthfully denied the possible sources of worry suggested by the first physician because his line of questioning did not lead him to see himself in the way that the second physician's questioning did. The differences, although subtle, are fundamental to success in talking with a patient. The second physician's history had been productive because his

> *"The physician must understand the significance to the patient of his or her life events."*

questions were open-ended, brief, sympathetic, and thought-provoking. The patient, by telling about himself in his own words, provided the leads to where his trouble lay.

As Sir William Osler said, "It is more important to know what kind of patient has the disease than what kind of disease the patient has." A life story means little as a recital of events unless the physician understands the peculiar significance of the events to the particular patient concerned. Much of this information cannot be gathered from answers to direct questions. Rather, it must be inferred from the patient's account of his life story, the organization of his lifestyle, and the kinds of decisions that he has made. The details of the events themselves are important only if they indicate something about the person by the way in which they were handled. One cannot tell much about a piece of music by simply knowing what notes were used. Rather, it is the arrangement of the notes, the timing, the modulations, and the emphases that convey meaning to the listener. Similarly, a simple account of unfortunate events and conflicts, together with emotional responses to them, may be only marginally helpful. A limited number of emotional conflicts plague almost everyone to some degree at some time or other. The significant information lies in the attitude or *Weltanschauung* of the patient, his or her view of the world and his or her way of perceiving and dealing with it. To achieve a level of dialogue productive of such information requires a highly developed intuition and ability to adapt one's speech and manner to the circumstances and experience of the patient, and to his or her intellectual level and sociocultural background.

The social background and the subculture in which the patient grew up can yield important data to a physician familiar with ethnic and regional attitudes and customs. For example, Miss G., a 26-year-old Italian-American woman, complained of nausea and vomiting so troublesome and incapacitating that she could not work. As the story unfolded, it developed that she was unmarried. The physician was able to detect an incongruity and a potential source of conflict by virtue of his familiarity with the cultural patterns of first-generation Italian-Americans in New York City. If the patient had been a fifth-generation American who had attended a fashionable women's college, the fact that she was still unmarried would have had no significance. However, in the Italian culture in parts of New York City, it was customary to shield a girl from more than casual contacts with men until she was 18 years old, but to expect her to be married soon thereafter. Therefore, most young women reared in this culture are married well before the age of 26.

Beside being aware of social pressures and the cultural background, a knowledge of family values and personal aspirations may help the physician's understanding of his or her patient. Therefore, a broad liberal education and a varied life experience before entering medical school may be of great benefit to a physician in understanding and dealing with patients.

The Challenge to Medical Education

Today's entering medical students are considered generally to be better grounded in mathematics, biology, and chemistry than were their counterparts 20 or 30 years ago. In listening, writing, and speaking (the afferent and efferent aspects of communication), however, they are less well prepared. Ironically, in the medical experience of today there is less opportunity than before for students to learn the skills of dialogue from seasoned diagnosticians talking with patients on the wards and in the clinics.

The need to strengthen emphasis on communication in medical education poses a formidable challenge, but there are some hopeful signs on the horizon:

- Harvard Medical School's much touted "new" pathway mainly revives policies and practices prevalent among most leading medical schools in the United States before World War II. Nevertheless, this step backward appears to be a step forward.
- Organizations such as the American College of Physicians are urging third-party payers to recognize the importance of, and the need to compensate, physicians' time spent in talking with patients and in thoughtful analysis.
- Some still, small voices are calling for attention to poor physician-patient communications arising from fragmentation of responsibility for care among several physicians, excessive reliance on technology, and the tendency to substitute drug therapy for dialogue.

The Therapeutic Importance of Dialogue

Although the scope of this book does not include therapeutics, one cannot ignore the sometimes major therapeutic significance of talking with a skilled and understanding physician. Such an experience may enhance the effect of a prescribed medication or may by itself have an astonishing therapeutic effect, as in the case of Mr. S.

> *"Talking with an understanding physician may in itself have a beneficial effect."*

Illustrative Case

This patient was a 34-year-old television repairman whose previous physician had established the diagnosis of duodenal ulcer by radiography. He had been suffering from persistently recurring midepigastric pain and heartburn for five years, and since childhood he had been a stutterer. His mother had been an anxious, overprotective, and domineering woman. Mr. S. described his mother's behavior as follows:

> *Patient:*   She hated me to have magazines and a-a-a books, and I used to have to hide them under my s-s-s-sweater to get them into the house. Little

> things like that. And she didn't like my friends at all. I couldn't have
> them around, and she was always urging me to go to work. I hadn't
> even graduated from high school. I worked for a while, and I left
> home.

Physician: Why did she do it?

Patient: I think that she was a disturbed person, very much so . . . So I had a very harsh—I mean it was very hard for me, and that's one of the reasons I feel that my own s-s-son ought not to be a-a-a exposed to all that. Of course this is very ironic that a-a-a I married a woman who in s-s-s-some ways resembles her, but a-a-a . . .

Physician: In what way does she resemble her?

Patient: Well, in that she s-s-s-so often acts in an irrational way, a-a-a and she's aggressive.

Mr. S. then told of difficulties related to his speech impediment, of the poverty of his Russian-Jewish immigrant parents, and of his wife's higher social station. "My parents were always very, very poor, extremely poor; hers were a rung higher, awfully much higher."

He also told of his interest in art, literature, and philosophy, and of his having been a conscientious objector in World War II. In the course of the discussion he frequently expressed resentment of his wife and her rigid, domineering behavior.

The physician did very little but listen. Nevertheless, Mr. S. lost his epigastric symptoms, and he was not heard from for five months, at which time he was continuing to feel well. He had somehow managed to grasp the reins in his marital relationship. He had left his wife temporarily and had negotiated an agreement to return to her on the condition that he would be the head of the household. Mr. S. said, in a letter to the physician, "I've been able to eat anything without experiencing discomfort. It seems to me that my stomach is in better shape now than it has been in years. I've eaten highly spiced foods, fried and pickled foods, delicatessen, and so on, and have felt fine." Radiography and gastroscopy showed that the ulcer had healed without dietary or drug therapy.

Two months later Mr. S. wrote again:

> My wife accepted my terms and I went back to live with her. I've not regretted it.
> My wife has unquestionably changed, in an almost miraculous manner. I have
> been fairly easy-going with her and have not abused the authority I have de-
> manded. Whenever she has shown any signs of slipping back, however, I have
> reminded her that I meant business and would not tolerate any reversion to our
> old relationship. Our life together is in consequence no longer a constant battle
> for supremacy. Now that she has accepted my leadership, my wife tells me she is
> happier and far less tense. Others have commented on the change in her, too.

The following excerpt is from another letter written nine months after the original visit.

> The miracle of her personality change remains intact (it is incidentally the only
> miracle I have come in contact with).

Comment. Every contact with the patient has implications for treatment and, therefore, may have a favorable or unfavorable effect on the course of illness. The extraordinary power of words and feelings in a human relationship suggests that the physician may be the ultimate placebo.

Acknowledgment

I am indebted to Dr. Gordon H. Deckert, David Ross Boyd Professor of Psychiatry at the University of Oklahoma Health Sciences Center, for the illustrations and for advice and suggestions concerning the manuscript.

Suggested Reading

Bird B. Talking with patients. Philadelphia: JB Lippincott, 1955:154.

Byrne PS, Long BEL. Doctors talking to patients. London: Her Majesty's Stationery Office, 1976.

Cassell EJ. Talking with Patients. 2 vols. Cambridge: MIT Press, 1985:423.

Cutler P. Problem solving in clinical medicine. Baltimore: Williams & Wilkins, 1979:39.

Deckert GH, Andrews M. Interviewing techniques. In: Conn HF, Rakel RE, Johnson TW, eds. Family practice. Philadelphia: WB Saunders, 1978:258–266.

Deutsch F, Murphy WF. The clinical interview. New York: NY International University Press, 1960.

Enelow AJ, Swisher SN. Interviewing and patient care. New York: Oxford University Press, 1972.

Miller GA, Laird PN, et al. Language and perception. Cambridge: Belknap Press, 1976.

Osler W. Aequanimitas. With other addresses to medical students, nurses and practitioners of medicine. Philadelphia: Blakiston, 1943:451.

Raine CS, ed. Advances in neuroimmunology. New York: NY Academy of Sciences, 1988.

Richardson SA, Dohrenwend BS, Klein D. Interviewing. New York: Basic Books, 1965.

Wolf S. Talking with the patient. In: Bean WB, ed. Monographs in medicine. Baltimore: Williams & Wilkins, 1952:1–21.

Wolf S. The stomach. New York: Oxford University Press, 1965:321.

Wolf S. Abdominal diagnosis. Philadelphia: Lea & Febiger, 1979:209.

Wolf S. The stomach's link to the brain. Fed Proc 1985; 14:2889–2893.

Wolf S, Almy TP, Flynn JT, Kern F. Instruction in medical history taking. The use of wire and tape recorders. J Med Ed. 1952; 27:244–252.

Wolf S, Goodell HG, eds. Stress and disease. 2nd ed. Springfield: CC Thomas, 1968:277.

Wolf S, Goodell HG. Behavioral science in clinical medicine. Springfield: CC Thomas, 1976:230.

Wolf S, Wolff HG. Human gastric function: An experimental study of a man and his stomach. 2nd ed. New York: Oxford University Press, 1947:262.

Wolff HG, Wolf S, Hare C, eds. Life stress and bodily disease. Baltimore: Williams & Wilkins, 1950:1135.

ABDOMINAL PAIN

William S. Haubrich, M.D.

2

"Mankind are so accustomed to shrink from pain, and so eager in seizing upon every means to lessen or annul it, that the fact of our having been endowed with it, as with a sense, by a beneficent Creator, with the kindest intent, does not readily impress us."[1] This quotation, which appeared in the *Boston Medical and Surgical Journal* well over a century ago, prompts us to ponder that we have, indeed, been endowed with a sixth sense, apart from the five senses of sight, sound, smell, taste, and touch, whereby the faculty of pain warns us of impending danger or signals the presence of injury. Pain, despite its often being condemned as a cross mankind must bear, is in reality essential to life. One can be blind, deaf, insensitive to odor, bereft of taste, and lacking in tactile sense, yet still survive. Deprived of the ability to perceive pain, one is in grave peril. Wall makes the interesting and compelling point that pain is an awareness of need, like hunger, rather than awareness of event, like seeing or hearing.[2]

Moreover, pain, as much as we abhor it and as much as we strive to abolish it, is of prime importance, not only to the patient but also to his or her physician. Pain is often the key to diagnosis, which, in turn, opens the door to therapy. Bockus wrote: "The clinician who has a good understanding of pain mechanisms and is well trained in the interpretation of the many vagaries of abdominal pain has at hand the most important single aid in gastroenterologic diagnosis."[3]

To achieve an accurate diagnosis, it is essential that the physician systematically and painstakingly analyze the syndrome of pain as presented by each individual patient. A proper diagnosis requires an inductive approach. The astute physician begins with the particulars, evident in symptoms and signs, and then works methodically toward a logical conclusion, which is tantamount to a diagnosis. A tempting pitfall, of which the thoughtful physician is wary, is to postulate a hasty diagnosis and then insistently cram bits of information into a narrow category, simply to conform to a preconceived label.

Lest these remarks asserting the benefit of pain be misconstrued, I hasten to point out that this chapter is not intended as a paean to pain. As helpful as it can be, pain also has its downside. Pain, particularly when unrelenting and unrelieved, is a trying burden to the sufferer and can, in itself, be deleterious. This is all the more reason why pain should be carefully assessed and properly appreciated so that, once its useful function has been served, pain can be effectively allayed.

Pain, of course, is more than a mere sensation. The experience of pain includes (1) *nociception,* the registration of a noxious stimulus and instigation of an impulse conveying a signal of hurt or injury; (2) *perception* of the painful sensation; (3) *distress,* in terms of a negative affective response; and (4) *behavior,* directed or misdirected, consequent to the perception of pain and the distress it induces. All of these components must be taken into account when attempting to assess the patient's complaint of pain. Collectively, these components involve almost the entire nervous system of the organism, from minute receptors at the periphery, along afferent nerve tracks, through various modifying stations in the spinal cord and brain stem, and on to the highest centers in the brain itself.

Anatomy of Abdominal Pain

Receptors

Most, but not all, pain impulses begin with activation of neuroreceptors. Those receptors capable of responding to noxious stimuli are known as nociceptors (Fig. 2–1). Pain of central origin, sometimes called "psychogenic pain," will be dealt with later. Neuroreceptors are situated throughout the abdominal viscera and their supporting structures. Receptors of stimuli that give rise to pain are not so numerous or sensitive in abdominal viscera as are their counterparts in the skin, but they are present. Also, visceral nociceptors do not usually generate impulses by stimuli that would excite cutaneous receptors. For example, it has long been known that the intact mucosa of the alimentary tract is insensitive to pricking, cutting, or crushing, stimuli that would be expected to cause sharp pain if applied to the skin. For this reason, endoscopic biopsy specimens can be plucked from the gastrointestinal mucosa without anesthesia, the patient unaware of any discomfort owing to the procedure. Polyps can be painlessly snared and exercised. A heat probe, an electrocoagulator, or even a laser beam can be applied to the alimentary mucosa with no painful sensation perceived by the patient. The striking difference in sensitivity of skin and mucosa is clearly

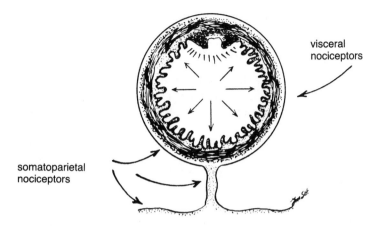

FIGURE 2-1.   Visceral nociceptors situated in the wall of a hollow viscus responds mainly to changes in muscular tonus (i.e., hypertonicity), as in either spasm or distention, and to ischemia. An injured or inflamed mucosa also can give rise to visceral pain impulses. Somatoparietal nociceptors situated in the peritoneum and mesentery respond to stretching, tugging, and inflammation.

evident in the anorectal segment. The columnar-lined mucosa, even within a few millimeters of the dentate or pectinate line, can be attacked by biopsy forceps, snare, or coagulator with impunity. But barely a millimeter or so on the other side of the line, where the lining is stratified squamous epithelium (i.e., skin), the same procedure would elicit howls of anguish from the patient. Woe betide the careless examiner (and his or her hapless patient) who mistakes a hypertrophied anal papilla for an adenomatous polyp and attempts to uproot it!

An inflamed or otherwise injured mucosa, however, is another matter. Pain can arise from an inflamed alimentary mucosa, probably because of a sensitizing effect on neuroreceptors by nocireactive substances elaborated in response to injury. Minute, superficial erosions in columnar epithelium typically are painless, but pain can be felt in deeper, edematous, and inflamed ulcerations. Infiltration by neoplasia, unfortunately, often is painless in its beginning stages, and the patient is thereby deprived of what otherwise might be an early warning of the lesion.

There are stimuli of other sorts that can give rise to discomfort, even intense pain, in the viscera. Receptors in the wall of the alimentary tract can be keenly sensitive to changes in tonus, either tight contraction or ballooning distention. Contraction or distention in segments of the alimentary tract, as occurs in the process of normal digestion, do not usually cause a disagreeable sensation (else each one of us would be miserable after every ordinary meal). However, both forceful contraction of smooth muscle, as can occur when the gut is trying to overcome a point of obstruction, and the marked distention that can occur proximal to an obstruction can give rise to pain.

Moreover, even the intact and relaxed gut is liable to respond painfully to tugging, stretching, or pulling. This incites pain receptors in the mesentery and the root by which it is attached to the peritoneum. There is also an appreciable difference in sensitivity that distinguishes the serosal and parietal peritoneal surfaces. This is clearly evident at laparoscopy. The tip of the endoscope or a probe can gently prod the serosal surface of the gut and elicit little or no painful response in the unanesthetized patient; the same light touch or abrasion of the parietal surface is keenly felt.

In addition, the abdominal viscera can be painfully responsive to ischemia, consequent to arterial atherosclerosis, thrombosis, or embolism. Fortunately, most of the viscera are favored by abundant collateral circulation. Thus, while abrupt deprivation of blood supply can be acutely painful, gradual and protracted impairment is less often so. Even when collateral circulation fails, the gut at rest is relatively painless, but when the patient attempts to ingest food and the metabolic need for increased arterial circulation is unmet, the gut writhes in agony. This is the visceral pain of arterial mesenteric insufficiency.

It helps to know, then, when analyzing a patient's reported pain or when conducting procedures on an unanesthetized patient, where pain receptors are located and how they can be expected to respond to a particular stimulus.

Transmission

Much has been learned of the means by which afferent impulses originating by stimulation of pain receptors find their way to successively higher centers in the nervous system, where they are registered, sorted out, and modulated (Fig. 2–2). Although much remains to be learned of this intricate process, we know enough to intelligently approach the problem of pain.

Suffice it to say here that pain impulses, once generated, can travel along either or both of two types of afferent fibers: (1) large, thinly myelinated fibers given to quick conduction (12 to 80 meters per second), responding to tactile, thermal, or chemical stimuli, and conveying discriminative information related to the location and intensity of the stimuli; and (2) small, unmyelinated fibers given to slower conduction (0.4 to 1.0 meter per second), responding to stimuli arising in tissue injury, and conveying "hurt" without telling exactly where or what it is. The larger fibers (called A-delta fibers) conduct impulses that are registered as *epicritic* (i.e., enabling acute sensitivity). The smaller fibers (called C fibers) conduct impulses that are *protopathic* (i.e., conveying a more general, basic sense of injury).

It is a competition between impulses transmitted along these differing fibers, both of which can be activated simultaneously, that gives rise to the "gate theory" proposed by Melzack and Wall.[4] According to this postulate, if input conveyed by the large fiber predominates, then an inhibitory neuron prevails, and the "gate" is shut; the message of pain is suppressed. If, however, the stimulus is sufficiently intense, then input conveyed by the smaller fiber pre-

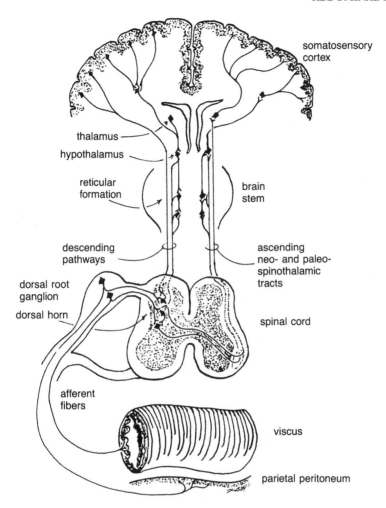

somatosensory
cortex

thalamus

hypothalamus

reticular
formation

brain
stem

descending
pathways

ascending
neo- and paleo-
spinothalamic
tracts

dorsal root
ganglion

dorsal horn

spinal cord

afferent
fibers

viscus

parietal peritoneum

FIGURE 2–2. Simplified scheme showing afferent pathways from the viscera and peritoneum, through the spinal cord, and ascending, by way of modulating centers, to the sensory cortex of the cerebrum. Descending pathways also modulate pain perception and response to pain.

vails; the inhibitory neuron is suppressed, and the message of pain comes through loud and clear. This could help to explain certain well-known homely responses to pain; for example, rubbing the skin over the part that hurts. It could explain the benefit, long-held but nowadays sometimes forgotten, of applying hot stupes to a sore belly. On a more up-to-date, high-tech level, the theory could justify the use of a transcutaneous electrical stimulator to allay pain.

Impulses carried by both large and small afferent fibers converge on cell bodies in the dorsal root ganglia and thence to synapses in the dorsal horn of the spinal cord. Recent investigation indicates that the dorsal horn is a more complex structure, in terms of afferent transmission, than was once thought. The dorsal horn has been found to contain intrinsic neurotransmitter peptides, such as enkephalins and substance P, that can modify impulses brought to the spinal cord from the periphery. The dorsal horn is not a mere synaptic way-station. Rather, it plays an essential role in deciding which impulses to cancel out, which impulses to deal with by efferent response at the segmental spinal cord level, and which impulses to convey to higher centers.

Those impulses destined for higher centers are transmitted to second-order relay neurons. The axons of these neurons then cross to the contralateral spinal cord and begin their ascent along the spinothalamic tracts, terminating in either the reticular formation in the brain stem, or higher yet in the hypothalamus and thalamus. From there, third-order neurons convey impulses to the limbic system and the somatosensory cortex of the cerebrum, which constitute neurologic substrates of pain perception and pain-related behavior. Various neuroregulatory peptide substances recently have been recognized to play a modifying role also in these higher centers.[5] There is no known, discrete "pain center."

This three-tiered, three-neuron ascending afferent system is by no means all there is to the total "pain experience." Descending tracts from the cerebral cortex connect with neurons in the brain stem and thence to the dorsal horn, where neurotransmitting substances, chiefly serotonin, are capable of modulating or inhibiting responses to pain sensation.

> *"Higher centers of the brain influence how pain is perceived and how reaction to pain is manifest."*

It has long been debated whether pain (or whatever might be perceived as pain in the abdomen or elsewhere in the periphery) can originate within a disturbed area of the brain itself, in the absence of an outlying stimulus. So-called "central pain" is not pain merely imagined but pain actually felt in the abdomen, yet wholly unprovoked by any disturbance in the abdominal wall or its contents. The debate is far from settled, and the question remains arguable. There is yet to be demonstrated a discrete cerebral or brain stem lesion that in itself gives rise to abdominal pain simulating intra-abdominal disease or injury. There are, of course, lesions of the spinal cord and its neural appendages that can cause pain referred to the periphery. A ground on which most, if not all, clinicians can agree is that varying conditions pertaining in higher centers of the brain undoubtedly influence the intensity at which pain, otherwise stimulated, is perceived and how reaction to a given pain is manifest. Most clinicians can testify to their encounters with "pain-prone" persons whose tortuous narratives of past and present complaints support a conviction that they are endowed with a keenly sensitive nervous system.[6] On the other hand, perhaps we might all be "pain-prone," given sufficiently conducive circumstances.

Appreciation of Abdominal Pain

All of this seems awesomely complicated, yet the actual appreciation of abdominal pain can be simplified if one thinks in terms of three afferent relays or pathways for pain impulses:

1. *Visceral or splanchnic pathways* activated by nociceptors situated in the walls or substance of the abdominal viscera.
2. *Somatic or parietal pathways* activated by nociceptors situated in the parietal peritoneum and supporting tissues.
3. *Referral pathways* activated by strong visceral impulses "spilling over" to somatic afferent neurons in the same spinal cord segment.

None of these pathways are mutually exclusive, and often they act in concert, although the visceral and somatic pathways may operate independently (Table 2–1).

With this triad in mind, we can then think in terms of what might be called (1) visceral pain, (2) somatic or parietal pain, and (3) referred pain.

Visceral Pain. Visceral pain tends to be felt as a dull soreness, but at times can be intense; it tends to waver or fluctuate in severity; it is vaguely or poorly localized, usually felt in the midline regardless of the anatomic situation of its stimulus; it may be described by the patient as aching, cramping, gnawing, or burning, or sometimes not as pain at all but rather as a disagreeable "all-gone" feeling; often it is perceived as a "sick pain" (i.e., attended by restlessness, nausea, vomiting, sweating, pallor, and such symptoms concomitant with autonomic efferent disturbance).

TABLE 2–1. Distinguishing Characteristics of Visceral and Somatoparietal Pain

Visceral Pain	Somatoparietal Pain
Dull	Sharp
Wavering	Sustained
Poorly localized (referred to midline)	Focal (indicates site of stimulus)
Induces restlessness	Prompts immobility
Attended by other symptoms of autonomic disturbance	Usually stands out alone
May be described in terms other than "pain"	Usually perceived clearly as "pain"

Somatic or Parietal Pain.   Somatic or parietal pain tends to be more acute, more intense, and more likely to be sustained; it is more sharply localized, usually indicating the anatomic site of its stimulus; it tends to be aggravated by movement, so that the patient is inclined to lie still. While hardly agreeable, somatic pain, in unusual circumstances, can be almost exhilarating. An example might be the soldier who sustains "a million-dollar wound," exempting him from the anguish of further combat. Persons who have experienced both visceral and somatic pain, and have distinguished their features, profess to opt for somatic rather than visceral pain, if pain would have to be experienced again.

Referred Pain.   Referred pain combines features of both visceral and somatic pain; it tends to be fairly well localized in areas remote from the inciting stimulus, yet supplied by the same neural segment as the injured organ; often it is attended by cutaneous or muscular hyperesthesia in the area of referral. Occasionally, the sensation of pain in the referred area predominates, and the inciting visceral pain is subdued and hardly mentioned, or even forgotten by the patient.

How these different pathways interact in clinical circumstances is described in the later exposition of specific examples of abdominal pain.

Attributes of Abdominal Pain

Duration.   The duration of pain often is the first clue to its significance. As with most symptoms, there is an inverse relation between the length of time that pain has been experienced and the likelihood that pain can be traced to a particular lesion. The search for the cause of acute pain of short duration, especially that which can be dated to a recent day or hour, is much more likely to be rewarded by finding and identifying its stimulus than is a pain that the patient says "has always been there." I remember the day when a frail old lady tottered into my office and, before I had a chance to greet her, informed me, "Doctor, I'm 80 years old, and I've been sick every day of my life." I confess my attention was blunted as I listened to her long tale of woe. I doubted that subsequent examination would reveal a clear-cut cause of her misery, and my doubt was later confirmed. On the other hand, the patient who says, "I didn't know I had a stomach until that pain struck last night" sends a more compelling message. Pain of long duration can by no means be dismissed or ignored, but pain of short duration is more liable to explanation.

Mode of Onset.   The mode of onset can be significant. The more abrupt (and least expected) the onset, the easier will be the task of pinpointing its origin in most cases. Acute pain of sudden onset and high intensity suggests an intra-abdominal catastrophe, either mechanical, as in perforation or obstruction, or vascular, as in abrupt occlusion of a blood vessel. Pain of gradual onset is the more common mode, and here the incidence of crescendo may be helpful. Pain of very slow increase in intensity suggests a beginning in a smoldering lesion; pain of rapid increase in intensity suggests a quickly evolving lesion.

Intermittency. Intermittency (or lack thereof) of pain is worthy of note. Acute pain that comes and goes, but with symptom-free intervals of short or long duration, usually signifies a remittent, then recurrent, lesion or injurious condition. Typical are the symptom-free intervals that separate acute bouts of biliary tract pain. Mention has been made that pain impulses traversing visceral or splanchnic pathways tend to be wavering if not intermittent, whereas pain impulses conveyed by parietal pathways tend to be more sustained. Few abdominal lesions give rise to unremitting, unrelenting, constant pain of unending duration.

Intensity. Intensity of pain, as perceived by the patient, is often difficult, if not impossible, for the physician to address. One is obliged to take the patient's word for how much it hurts. There are, however, clues in attending symptoms and signs and in the manner by which the patient describes his or her pain. Once in a while one encounters an incredibly stoic patient who may be admitted in shock with a board-like abdomen. "Does it hurt?" seems like a foolish question, but even more surprising is the patient's reply—"Not really."

There are patients whose experience with pain is limited, so that they may lack a point of reference and have little basis for comparison. Comparison can be revealing. The woman who says "This pain is worse than any I ever felt with childbirth," is probably suffering intense pain. Then there are persons who are habituated to describing every sensation with hyperbole. A hangnail is "excruciating." The soreness of a twisted ankle prompts, "I thought I'd die!" Stranger still is the patient who appears relatively impassive while describing pain in terms of exceeding intensity, a seeming paradox dubbed "la belle indifférence"—distress described in a setting of apathy.

One may be tempted to ask the patient to rate the perceived intensity of pain on a scale of 1 to 10. This is not usually helpful when applied to a single episode of pain, but it may be useful in judging variance in pain when one episode is compared with another.

Much has been made of what has been called "pain threshold," based on an assumption that persons differ according to the strength of stimulus required to elicit a sensation of pain. According to this concept, some persons have a high threshold for pain and hence are relatively insensitive, whereas others have a low threshold for pain and therefore respond to even the slightest painful stimulus. Evidence for differing thresholds of sensation is lacking in most studies of the problem. In experimental conditions, a majority of persons become aware that a potentially painful stimulus has been applied at a fairly uniform level of intensity. What differs from one person to another is the graded level of a given stimulus that induces a response of distress. If this is true, then perhaps we should think in terms of thresholds of reaction rather than pain thresholds.

It should not be necessary to point out that what is judged to be the intensity of a given patient's pain cannot be used to distinguish "functional" from "organic" disorders. Patients exhibiting what can only be described as functional disturbances not infrequently perceive intense abdominal pain: conversely, there are patients harboring extensive and pervasive organic lesions who perceive relatively little pain.

Finally, I can state that in many years of clinical practice (including a few years of military duty), I have rarely encountered true malingering. From my own experience, few have been those patients who straight-facedly complained of pain when, in fact, they knowingly perceived no pain at all.

"We should think in terms of thresholds of reaction rather than pain thresholds."

Pain is essentially a private matter. It has been aptly said that the patient perceives pain but doesn't know what to do about it; the physician knows what to do about pain but can only surmise what the patient feels.

Site. Localization, depth, and radiation of pain as indicated by the patient can be both helpful and misleading. It is important to remember that stimuli within the abdomen can give rise to pain perceived elsewhere. In assessing symptoms of abdominal disease or injury, as Sir William Osler observed, the abdomen must be thought of as extending from the neck to the knees. For example, a lesion under either hemidiaphragm may give rise to shoulder-top pain, moreover, the shoulder-top pain may predominate over pain perceived at or below the level of the diaphragm. The pain of a pancreatic lesion classically is referred to the back. A stimulus to pain in the cecum or sigmoid colon may be perceived as pain in either hip or thigh or in the lower back (Fig. 2–3).

Mention has been made that pain transmitted solely along visceral afferent pathways tends to be poorly localized and to be referred to the midline regardless of the lateral location of the stimulus. In general, the level of midline pain can be a clue. Pain from the hepatobiliary structures and from the alimentary tract proximal to the ligament of Treitz tends to be felt in the epigastrium; pain from the small bowel tends to be periumbilical; and pain from the colon tends to be felt in the lower abdomen.

Patients usually can distinguish between deep and superficial pain. However, a problem here is that referred pain often is associated with cutaneous hyperesthesia. For example, the distress of uncomplicated peptic ulcer usually is felt

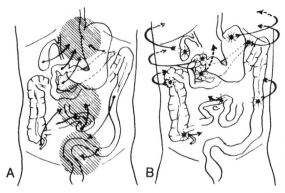

FIGURE 2-3. *A*, Approximate levels at which visceral pain typically is felt; *B*, more sharply localized foci of somatoparietal pain and common sites of extension.

in the epigastrium, but it may be attended by such epigastric skin sensitivity that a lesion in the subcutaneous abdominal wall might be suspected.

It is always helpful to ask the patient to indicate with his or her own hand where it hurts. It is helpful, too, to observe how the patient does this. If the patient uses an outstretched palm to make vague, sweeping gestures hither and yon over the abdomen, not much can be learned of the site of the painful stimulus. But if the patient makes a single, deliberate gesture with an extended index finger, that one spot, especially when associated with focal tenderness,

> "**A**sk the patient to indicate with his or her own hand where it hurts."

may be the source of the problem. There is, however, an important exception: the distress of peptic ulcer typically is localized to a finger-tip point; the ulcer may be duodenal and thus situated well to the right of the midline and below the rib margin, but the patient points toward the xiphoid process. In the case of a postoperative marginal or anastomotic ulcer, the patient is more likely to point to a shift of pain away from the midline.

Character. The character of perceived pain should be helpful in tracing its source, but often it is not. While the patient should always be encouraged to describe pain in his or her own words, the vocabulary of the average patient is not richly endowed with distinctive terms for various kinds of pain or distress. The average patient knows only that it hurts. But the same patient can be prompted to a finer distinction, if the examiner, by suggesting various descriptive terms, is careful to avoid leading questions. Usually the patient responds by

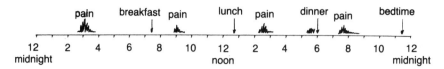

FIGURE 2-4. Constructing a simple diurnal time chart can be helpful in relating pain or distress to circumstances.

describing the pain in terms such as "like an ache," "like a knot being tied," or "like burning" (Fig. 2-4). A sensation of "burning" is often a *forme fruste* of pain, being related, to borrow Longfellow's phrase, "as the mist resembles the rain."

The patient's previous experience with pain of various types is sometimes helpful. It is interesting to observe that even a relatively inarticulate patient can make an accurate distinction between differing types of pain. The patient may not be able to tell exactly how he or she makes the distinction, but he or she knows there is a difference. If the patient says, "This is not like the pain I had with my kidney stone," the chances are that his or her present pain is not due to

"The patient may describe pain as burning, piercing, gnawing, boring, bloating, cramping, gripping, or fluttering."

recurrent nephrolithiasis. But here again, a word of caution: one has to allow for evolution in a given lesion. For example, the patient may be well acquainted with ordinary, uncomplicated peptic ulcer distress, but the pain felt when that ulcer has deeply penetrated into the pancreas is quite different.

There is yet another problem familiar to all clinicians, and that is encountered in the patient who insists in describing his or her pain in terms of diagnosis. Such utterances as "My ulcer has been acting up right here" or "My gallbladder pain is right there" may be accurate or may be misleading. The fact is, of course, that neither the patient nor the physician should jump to a premature diagnostic conclusion until the particular pain has been carefully assessed.

Relation to Alimentary Function. Noting the temporal relation of pain to alimentary function can be of prime importance in assaying the cause of abdominal pain. Especially informative can be remarks such as "It hurts only when I try to swallow" or "If I eat a little something, the pain goes away but then comes back after an hour or so" or "If I don't eat or drink anything, then I have no cramps." For remittent and recurrent pain through the day, construction of a simple diurnal chart may be helpful (see Fig. 2–4). Better yet, ask the patient to keep a diary, noting the times of meals along with the timing and duration of pain. It is surprising how often a temporal association between eating and pain is at first unappreciated by the patient, only to find that a distinct relationship becomes evident when daily events are recorded. Of importance here is the relation of pain to the time of eating, not necessarily to what has been eaten. Mostly myth is the notion that a fatty meal always provokes biliary tract pain. Nor is it true that spicy foods invariably aggravate acid-peptic distress.

Relation to Extra-alimentary Events. Important, too, is charting a relation to extra-alimentary circumstances. Extrinsic conditions preceding or concurrent with the noxious stimulus plays a telling role in the perception of pain. Abdominal pain or distress is influenced by the coincident mental milieu at the time that visceral or parietal nociceptors are triggered. On a day when the patient is beset by intense headache or emotional upheaval, abdominal pain, when stimulated, is bound to be perceived as more intense than on a day when conditions are otherwise tranquil. Anger has been shown to intensify perception of abdominal pain.[7] All of this is part of what has been called the "psychic signature" of pain. C.S. Sherrington, many years ago, referred to the relation of emotion and pain as "the psychic adjunct of an imperative protective reflex."[8]

Preceding or concurrent physical or emotional stress is noteworthy, of course. However, in this regard one should be mindful of the paradoxical "garrison syndrome," which first became evident in military medicine. One might think the strain of battle would be greatest for a soldier when he is precariously positioned on the fighting line. This is not always the case. Sometimes the effect of stress becomes apparent only when the soldier is withdrawn from the heat of combat and sheltered in the relative safety of a behind-the-lines garrison. No longer sustained by the excitement of battle, the soldier "falls apart."

I have seen the counterpart of the garrison syndrome in civilian life. I remember a gracious, middle-aged lady who was suffering from a painfully irritable bowel. When inquiry was made of a possibly provocative stress, she was perplexed. Yes, she had been the victim of stress. For a number of months she had been obliged to nurse her aged mother in the throes of terminal cancer. The mother's eventual death, while expected, was still a shock. Then there was the ordeal of settling her mother's affairs. Stress she had had in abundance. But during the stress of nursing and mourning, she had felt little if any abdominal discomfort. It was only when her grief had passed and she had resumed what seemed a more tranquil existence that she found herself suffering from a painful bowel.

The mental milieu that most commonly intensifies or prolongs the anguish of pain is depression.[9] When assessing the possible influence of a depressed state, it is helpful to inquire of other features characteristic of depression. Has appetite declined? Has sleep been elusive? Is the capacity for concentration diminished? Has the patient lost interest in usually absorbing activities? Have there been seemingly unprovoked bouts of "the blues" or of unaccustomed weeping?

A diurnal pattern of pain is worth noting, aside from a relation to alimentary function. As every seasoned clinician knows, pain occurring at night can be particularly disagreeable. In part, this is because of the ominous aura of dismal darkness; in part, it is because of the lack of distraction by daytime activity. Occurrence of pain during the night suggests but does not necessarily indicate a specific "organic" stimulus. In cases of night pain, it is important to ask whether pain actually rouses the patient from sleep or whether the patient finds himself unable to sleep and then becomes aware of pain. If pain is present at bedtime, does it prevent the patient from falling asleep? If pain seems to awaken the patient in the morning, is it at the usual time of getting up or is it earlier?

Circadian rhythms, aside from those governing mealtimes, also can influence the course of abdominal pain. Susceptibility to abdominal distress is likely to be heightened when established rhythms are disturbed, as by changing work shifts or by jet travel.[10] Recently, functional abdominal pain has been associated with 6-sulfatoxy melatonin and with temperature rhythms of low amplitude, presumably because of suppression of circadian oscillators.[11]

Beyond a diurnal pattern, one looks for relationships on a longer span. Is pain greater or less during the work week or during the leisure of weekends? Have periods of vacation altered the occurrence or intensity of pain? In premenopausal women, is pain consistently related to menses? For many women, abdominal distress from any cause is aggravated during the premenstrual phase.[12]

Essential to an assessment of pain is an accurate recording of medications or drugs taken by the patient before, during, and after a bout of distress. Have the symptoms been a recognized side effect of medications taken for another purpose? Have drugs possibly aggravated or perhaps ameliorated abdominal pain? Have the type and dose of analgesics been appropriate for the pain described?

It is important to note the relation of pain to activity and posture. Mention has been made that abdominal pain transmitted along visceral afferent pathways tends to be attended by restlessness; the patient, then, in the throes of visceral pain, tends to twist and turn, to move about and pace the floor. When parietal receptors and pathways are invoked, the patient prefers to remain quietly at rest.

It can be instructive to ask the patient to demonstrate, in the examining room or in the hospital bed, the postures that he or she has found to aggravate or to relieve pain. How posture can affect pain is related in some of the following clinical examples.

Clinical Examples of Digestive Tract Pain

Esophageal Pain

Pain from lesions of the esophagus generally is felt retrosternally and often is referred to the interscapular area of the back. Usually the level at which pain is perceived is related to the level of the lesion. For example, pain from a lesion in the upper third of the esophagus typically is felt in the region of the suprasternal notch; pain from a lesion in the midesophagus tends to be felt beneath the midsternum; and pain from a lesion in the lower esophagus is felt at the xiphisternal junction. However, there is one important disclaimer to this generalization. Lesions in the lower esophagus or at the esophagogastric junction often induce secondary hypertonicity in the upper esophageal sphincter. This reflex contraction may lead the patient to complain of pain in the lower throat, distant from the primary lesion.

Pain emanating from the esophagus typically is characterized as a burning sensation. This, along with a vague reference to the midchest, is what would be expected of esophageal pain, insofar as the esophagus is endowed with nociceptors serving the visceral afferent pathways. The esophagus differs from the rest of the alimentary tract in not being invested by a serosa; therefore, the esophagus has no parietal receptors of its own. Unless an esophageal lesion has penetrated the mediastinum to the pleura or pericardium, esophageal pain is not sharply localized.

Of course, one must distinguish between the distress of dysphagia and the actual pain of odynophagia (see Chapter 4, "Swallowing Problems: Dysphagia and Odynophagia"). This distinction may be difficult for the patient to convey. Dysphagia and odynophagia by no means always coincide; in fact, the two symptoms are usually exclusive. A carcinoma occluding the lumen of the esophagus is manifest predominantly as difficulty in swallowing. Carcinoma confined to the esophageal wall is attended by little or no pain. Later, when an infiltrating carcinoma extends to adjacent structures or prevents accommodative distention of the esophagus, pain is added to dysphagia. On the other hand, acute mucosal inflammation in the esophagus can be evident by pain on swallowing when there is no compromise of the esophageal lumen and no actual dysphagia. In either case, the patient is reluctant to eat, but for different reasons.

One of the most frequent dilemmas confronting the clinician is posed by the patient with chest pain, and the question is whether the pain is of cardiac or esophageal origin. Almost always it is cardiac pain that is thought of first by the patient and initially considered by the primary physician. When cardiac pain presumably has been excluded, the clinician is asked to establish that the esophagus is the source of chest pain. This is often difficult to do, but there are, however, symptomatic distinctions. Esophageal pain seldom extends to the jaw or arms but can be referred to the interscapular area. The most important distinction of esophageal pain when compared with cardiac pain is its relation to activity and posture. Cardiac pain, especially that due to coronary arterial insufficiency, typically is aggravated by exertion and relieved by rest; esophageal pain is not. Esophageal pain, especially that related to gastroesophageal reflux, typically is provoked by stooping, crouching, and recumbency; in contrast, recumbency tends to relieve cardiac pain.

The most frequent expression of "heartburn" is by the patient with hiatus hernia of the common axial or sliding type; patients with hiatus hernia of the para-esophageal type seldom complain of "heartburn" (see Chapter 4). Burning distress can be, and often is, caused by esophageal spasm, but usually it also signifies reflux into the esophagus or irritating acid-peptic stomach contents, which can induce sharp contraction of the esophagus. Clearly, gastroesophageal reflux has occurred when the patient complains of "acid brash" (i.e., a welling up in the throat of bitter, sour fluid). When the patient unmistakably describes acid brash, there is no need for cumbersome, invasive tests to prove that fluid of low pH is encroaching on the esophagus. A patient who is habitually awakened by mouthfuls of acid gastric juice together with burning retrosternal distress does not need overnight monitoring of his or her esophageal pH.

> *"The single most important question is whether heartburn occurs only during the day or disturbs sleep at night."*

A variant is "bile brash," a regurgitation of bitter gall that is less likely to be attended by retrosternal pain. This may indicate dysfunction both at the pylorus and at the lower esophageal sphincter. The symptom is often encountered in patients who have had previous pyloroplasty or gastric resection. Even more startling is fecal regurgitation by a patient with gastrocolic fistula.

Occasionally, a patient will mention "water brash" (i.e., a usually painless welling up of tasteless fluid in the throat or mouth). This is not significant of acid reflux but rather is due to either an outpouring of mucus secretion from the esophagus or hypersalivation resulting from subliminal nausea, or both. Water brash can be a signal of subliminal nausea (see Chapter 5, "Nausea and Vomiting").

The single most important question to ask the patient complaining of heartburn or acid brash is whether the symptom occurs when sitting upright during daytime or whether it disturbs his or her sleep when recumbent at night. Some patients, of course, will say both. The distinction is that occasional, mild heartburn or acid brash occurring shortly after meals is a common experience, even in the absence of hiatus hernia. The symptoms may be significant of acid-peptic reflux, which can occur normally, but in this circumstance the esophagus usually clears itself rapidly of the irritating fluid, and little or no damage is done. Nocturnal gastroesophageal reflux, however, is often not so readily cleared, and the noxious fluid is more likely to induce mucosal injury. Postprandial heartburn can be an annoying nuisance and should be allayed; nocturnal acid brash is more likely to result in actual esophagitis and calls for further investigation and a more stringent remedy.

Peptic Ulcer Pain

Not all distress arising from peptic ulcer is "pain." Strangely, there are a few patients whose ulcer distress, in the absence of complication, is sufficient for them to seek medical help; yet they deny that they feel pain. These patients insist on describing an "empty stomach" discomfort or an "all-gone feeling." They may localize the feeling to a finger-tip area of the midepigastrium but repeatedly deny pain by that name. The symptom, if it follows a typical episodic, rhythmic pattern, is just as significant of ulcer activity as if it were called "pain."

More typical is a "burning" or "gnawing" pain pointedly localized in the midepigastrium or beneath the xiphoid process. Although pain of uncomplicated peptic ulcer disease is transmitted along visceral afferent pathways, this is an exception to the rule that visceral pain is only vaguely localized. As mentioned earlier, peptic ulcer pain typically is indicated by the patient, when asked to point to his or her pain, by the tip of an index finger.

Although almost invariably so localized, peptic ulcer pain is not always felt in the midepigastrium. I recall a patient who insisted that his ulcer pain was situated precisely at the left nipple and nowhere else. Another case, described by Dr. Tom Johnson, was that of a restaurant waiter whose ulcer pain was in a spot over his right shoulder. In both of these cases, the heterotopic pain was well localized and obeyed the rhythmic rule of the "pain–food–relief" sequence. Both cases were probably instances of unusual reference of pain (i.e., a "spilling over" of visceral impulses to afferent neurons serving an adjacent spinal cord segment).

In some cases of acid-peptic disease, epigastric cutaneous hypersensitivity is such that the patient complains of being unable to tolerate tight-fitting garments about the waist or of being unable to lean against a work table without discomfort.

In chronologic terms, the two principal features of peptic ulcer pain are *episodicity* and *rhythmicity*. Episodicity refers to the manner in which pain recurs in the long run of weeks, months, or years; rhythmicity refers to the manner in which pain recurs during a 24-hour cycle. Pain that is constantly unremitting or unrelenting can never be rightly ascribed to uncomplicated peptic ulcer disease. The patient who insists that his or her pain has never ceased through all the days of the past 5 years has thereby ruled out for the physician the possibility that the longstanding, unrelenting pain is caused by a peptic ulcer.

Episodicity.   Episodicity in peptic ulcer distress is sometimes mistakenly referred to as "periodicity." Episodes of symptomatically active peptic ulcer distress rarely occur periodically (i.e., at fixed and predictable intervals). A spell of ulcer distress is, by its nature, limited. Its intensity and duration vary from recurrence to recurrence, and the symptom-free intervals between episodes can vary, unpredictably, from weeks to months or even years. In the past, claims were made by some clinicians that episodes of ulcer activity tended to occur in the spring and fall, but I have not found that a seasonal occurrence, or lack thereof, is helpful in making a diagnosis of peptic ulcer disease. It seems to me that ulcer sufferers are as likely to complain of symptomatic bouts in the summer or winter as in the spring or fall.

> *"The keys to recognizing peptic ulcer distress are rhythmicity and episodicity."*

Neither have I found that bouts of ulcer pain in a given patient can be predicted to follow circumstances of notable stress. This is not to say that stress plays no role in peptic ulcer disease. I am simply saying that, in my experience, stress has not been an external factor that is consistently related to exacerbation of ulcer pain. There have been exceptions. One of my patients was an automotive engineer who invariably suffered recurrence of his peptic ulcer pain during November of every year. The explanation was that each November he was obliged to leave the familiar surroundings and regular schedule of his laboratory in Detroit and spend the month at an automotive test track in Arizona. Indeed, the month of testing involved long and grueling hours at the track, but I suspect another reason why his ulcer flared at such times was that his normal eating schedule was totally disrupted. At the track he was obliged to catch, if he could, a hasty gulp of food, but often he went hours with nothing at all in his stomach. Little wonder that his ulcer acted up at such a time.

Rhythmicity.   Rhythmicity is the next important key to recognizing peptic ulcer distress. This is the familiar sequence of pain–food–relief in the course of a given day. Peptic ulcers typically hurt when the stomach is empty; putting something (almost anything) in the stomach tends to allay ulcer pain, at least temporarily. Many patients claim milk as a favorite soother, but almost any food or fluid can yield some measure of relief. The interval of relative comfort after eating varies, probably dependent in part on the pace of stomach emptying. Some patients say that they can be assured of only a half-hour's relief after a meal; others say that they remain comfortable for several hours. But the sequence remains: pain–food–relief. Ulcer patients often are intolerant of delay at mealtime, and a productive question might be "Do you find yourself raiding the refrigerator to stave off hunger pangs?"

However, not all peptic ulcers, when active, give rise to this neat, rhythmic sequence. Consistent rhythmicity is most likely to be described by the patient whose ulcer is located at or near the pyloroduodenal junction. This, of course, encompasses that majority of patients whose peptic ulcers are situated in the duodenal bulb or cap. But the farther the ulcer is located away from the pylorus, either distally in the duodenum (rarely) or proximally in the stomach (commonly), the less one can rely on eliciting from that patient a well-defined pain–food–relief pattern.

Pain from gastric ulcers, especially those near the cardinal portion of the stomach, may be aggravated by eating. If one can elicit a history of a consistent pain–food–relief syndrome, this is a strong clue that the problem is pyloroduodenal; if such a history is not elicited, the presence of a peptic ulcer otherwise situated is not excluded.

One also must be cautious to avoid the snare of believing that a pain–food–relief syndrome invariably signifies the presence of an open, active peptic ulcer crater. The actual cause of peptic ulcer pain has long been debated, and the question has yet to be satisfactorily answered. There are those who hold that pain results mainly from spasm of the pyloroduodenal musculature; others have asserted vigorously that pain results rather from exposure of the ulcer crater to an acid pH. Both camps offer evidence favoring their assertions; both can cite evidence discounting the opposing view. Probably the truth lies in a middle ground embracing both mechanisms. Most clinicians believe that sufficiently intense pyloroduodenal contraction, even in the absence of an open ulcer crater, can give rise to ulcer-like pain. The point is that no syndrome, by itself, is pathognomonic for peptic ulcer. I recall that Dr. Henry L. Bockus, who was long concerned with the symptoms of peptic ulcer disease, never referred to a "peptic ulcer syndrome"; rather, he spoke of a "pyloroduodenal syndrome." His point, well-taken, is that occasionally one encounters a patient who describes an experience with pain or distress typical of peptic ulcer; yet neither radiography nor endoscopy has ever revealed an actual ulcer crater. This observation has been shared by all veteran clinicians. Dr. Bockus called this a "pseudo-ulcer syndrome" and attributed it to pyloroduodenal hypertonicity.

When asked what, other than food, might relieve their ulcer distress, patients often mention various antacids that many had tried before seeking professional advice. Common kitchen baking soda (sodium bicarbonate) used to be a folkloric favorite; nowadays, thanks to multimedia advertising, patients are more likely to have tried one or another of the proprietary nonabsorbable antacids. Relief of pain by antacids can be a clue, but the response is so nonspecific that it cannot be allowed as evidence of peptic ulcer disease. One cannot rely on a "therapeutic trial" for diagnosis.

Complications

What has been described thus far—episodes of well-localized midepigastric pain occurring in a rhythmic pattern—applies to uncomplicated gastroduodenal ulcers. Supervening complications of peptic ulcer disease alter the pattern of pain. The symptoms of complications that befall the patient with peptic ulcer—hemorrhage, obstruction, perforation—may or may not be preceded by a spell of typical ulcer pain. In some cases, the complication seems to strike "out of the blue," unheralded by any warning of ulcer activity. This circumstance has been described as a complication of a "silent ulcer." More often, if one presses the inquiry, some indication of precursory distress will be found. What might have been passed off as a "silent" ulcer may turn out to be one in which the milder, foregoing distress was forgotten in the alarm of complications.

It is not enough merely to ask the patient presenting with evidence of hemorrhage, obstruction, or perforation, "Have you ever had an ulcer?" A negative reply can be misleading. One should press further. I recall the following dialogue with a patient who for the first time sought medical care because of sudden, intense, abdominal pain and, when examined, was found to have a boardlike abdomen. An acute free perforation was obvious.

Physician: Have you ever had an ulcer?
Patient: No.
Physician: Have you ever had indigestion?
Patient: No.
Physician: Have you ever taken baking soda?
Patient: Oh, yes. At least a box a week.
Physician: Why?
Patient: To get rid of this misery in my stomach.

> **"I**t is not enough merely to ask the patient,
> 'Have you ever had an ulcer?'"

To me, this conversation was hard to explain, but it taught me to carry my questions beyond what might be thought necessary.

Hemorrhage.   Hemorrhage, when it occurs acutely and in copious quantity, usually but not always is preceded by a spell of fairly typical ulcer distress. When the stomach fills with exuded blood, pain tends to lessen and often disappears. Probably this is because the bolus of blood may inhibit py-loroduodenal spasm and also because blood is a buffer and tends to elevate the pH of the stomach contents. Slow oozing of blood from an ulcer crater has less effect on pain. The alarm of internal bleeding hastens intensive therapy with which pain ceases.

Obstruction.   Obstruction usually occurs at or near the pyloroduodenal junction and tends to be preceded by more or less typical ulcer pain. When pyloric stenosis leads to gastric stasis, the discomfort of the distended stomach is reflected first in cramping spasm, and then later in more vague, more steady epigastric distress. Any former pain–food–relief pattern is obscured. When stretching of the stomach wall has exceeded the capacity of its intrinsic smooth muscle to contract, the stomach loses tone and becomes a flaccid bag. There is no longer the cramping of spasm; there is only a vague feeling of disagreeable fullness.

Gastric stasis, of course, does not necessarily mean gastric outlet obstruction. The defect may be a loss of smooth muscle tonus in the gastric wall or some other motor dysrhythmia. This is not ordinarily a condition of peptic ulcer disease; rather, it is seen in neuromuscular disorders, the prime example being what is called "gastroparesis diabeticorum," a complication of longstanding diabetes mellitus. It is mentioned here because, in contrast to pyloric stenosis, this condition is remarkably painless. Probably this is because the neurovascular degeneration of advanced diabetes impairs afferent as well as efferent receptors and neural transmission.

Perforation.   Perforation appreciably alters the pattern of abdominal pain for the peptic ulcer patient, sometimes dramatically, sometimes more subtly. A distinction between the dramatic and the subtle derives from a distinction between acute free perforation and slower penetration with confined perforation.

The pain of *acute free perforation* strikes suddenly and reaches peak intensity almost immediately. Patients describe it as "like being kicked in the belly by a mule" (even though in this urban age mule kicks are uncommonly experienced, the simile remains apt). When gastric contents spill freely into the peritoneal cavity, severe pain is felt throughout the abdomen. As acidic, corrosive stomach fluid creeps under the domes of the diaphragm, pain may be referred to in the shoulders; as it trickles along the paraspinal gutters to the pelvis, it produces pain in the flanks and lower abdomen. There is an immediate reflex efferent stimulus to the muscles of the anterior abdominal wall. The consequently heightened tonus results in the characteristic "boardlike abdomen." If spillage is more of a seepage, and the seepage becomes contained in a smaller area, the pain, while intense, is more localized near the site of perforation, and muscular rigidity is limited in extent. When seepage is very slight, the condition is known as a forme fruste of acute free perforation.

It is pertinent here to comment on eliciting signs of peritoneal reaction. According to traditional teaching, the sign to be sought is that of "rebound tenderness." I would inveigh sternly against this teaching and proclaim that eliciting rebound tenderness should be banned from physical diagnosis. The reasons are these: first, if the sign is present, the maneuver is cruelly painful; second, the sign is not always reliable. If one depresses a distended, gas-filled, hollow viscus and then abruptly releases pressure, a sensitive patient may wince even though the bowel wall is intact. The mistaken impression may be that rebound tenderness has been elicited. Finally, there is a reliable yet humane maneuver that can be used to advantage in lieu of rebound tenderness. This is gentle palpation for underlying muscular rigidity. Some will argue that voluntary muscle contraction might be confused with the muscular rigidity of reflex peritoneal irritation; the experienced clinician will not be so confused. Sustained, involuntary muscular rigidity embodies all the significance of rebound tenderness with none of its harshness.

The change in ulcer pain by slow penetration and *confined perforation* is quite different from that of acute free perforation. In this complication, the ulcer crater and its surrounding inflammation have penetrated beyond the wall of the stomach or duodenum but have been confined or "walled off" by an adjacent structure or tissue. The most frequent circumstance is penetration of a posterior wall duodenal ulcer into the head of the pancreas. The patient is aware that something unusual has happened. Whereas his or her previous bouts of ulcer distress have followed the typical pain–food–relief sequence and the previous ulcer pain was well localized to the midepigastrium, now the pattern is distorted.

There are five cardinal, clinical features that betray the complication of confined perforation (Fig. 2–5): (1) extension of pain to the upper lumbar back, often so striking that one is prompted to think of the possibility of pancreatitis or pancreatic cancer; (2) supervention of night pain, particularly when nocturnal pain has not been a feature of uncomplicated ulcer distress; (3) a change in the location, spread, and intensity of anterior epigastric distress (what previously was finger-tip soreness in the midepigastrium becomes more widespread and more actually painful); (4) blurring of a formerly rhythmic pain–food–relief sequence (pain is more unrelenting and not so neatly related to meals); and (5) failure of relief by measures that previously allayed distress (a gulp of antacid no longer is soothing). All of these features are readily recognized when the appropriate questions are asked, and any or all can be indicative of the complication of confined perforation. The important point is to ask the patient how the current bout of distress compares with his or her previous experience.

It is sometimes said that vagotomy, as performed in the treatment of acid-peptic disease, will disturb or inhibit the registry of pain from a recurrent ulcer or will distort the pattern of pain that might otherwise be expected from any postoperative lesion in the upper abdomen. This is usually not the case. While

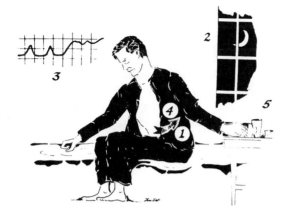

FIGURE 2-5. Evolving clinical features of complication of confined perforation are illustrated in this cartoon of a patient whose duodenal ulcer has penetrated deeply into the head of the pancreas. The altered symptoms (1–5) are described in the text.

the vagus nerve bears afferent fibers, few of these are involved in transmission of pain. A previous vagotomy does not, in most cases, alter the perception or pattern of abdominal pain provoked by any cause.

Small Bowel Pain

Lesions affecting the mesenteric small intestine typically give rise to pain felt in the midabdomen or the periumbilical area. When transmitted along visceral afferent pathways, pain is poorly localized and does not betray the anatomic site of the stimulus. In cases of mucosal inflammation or ulceration, pain tends to be felt as a deep soreness or ache; in cases of partial or complete intestinal obstruction, the pain of smooth muscle spasm tends to be cramping or colicky in nature.

It is curious that we often refer to any intermittent, acutely recurring, knotlike abdominal pain as "colic," a term often misapplied to biliary tract pain, as noted later. Colic obviously referred originally to the colon, but the small intestine is more liable to colicky pain than is the colon. The reason is that the small bowel is not normally disposed to distention and vigorously resists it; the large intestine is more accommodating to distention, which must reach an exaggerated proportion before the colon protests in pain.

Small bowel pain is usually aggravated by eating and allayed when the patient fasts.

It is only when a small bowel lesion, such as inflammation or neoplasia, extends through the serosa and affects the adjacent parietal peritoneum that parietal or somatic pain pathways are invoked. Then pain becomes more sharply localized to the site of the lesion and takes on more of the character of parietal pain.

The intestine is particularly sensitive to ischemia. Fortunately, the small intestine is seldom so affected, because of its rich blood supply and capacity for collateral circulation. However, when the supply of arterial blood from both the celiac axis and the superior mesenteric artery is curtailed, usually by atherosclerotic encroachment on the lumens of these major vessels near their origins, any alimentary burden thrust on the small bowel is met by intense pain, sometimes clumsily referred to as "abdominal angina." The pain eases when the bowel is idle. This furnishes a prime example for the setting of a symptom known as "sitophobia" (see Chapter 13, "Anorexia"). The patient can be ravenously hungry, yet declines food because its ingestion has been associated with extreme distress. Fortunately, pain caused by mesenteric arterial insufficiency, even in a patient otherwise ravaged by atherosclerosis, is relatively infrequent.

Colon Pain

Colon pain is similar to pain engendered in the small bowel and cannot be distinguished qualitatively. Colon pain differs in that it typically is felt in the lower reaches of the abdomen and, as mentioned above, is not so readily triggered by distention.

There is a syndrome peculiar to the colon that is related to gaseous distention of its hepatic and splenic flexures (see Chapter 12, "Gaseousness"). As an unusual anomaly, or sometimes as an acquired condition, the hepatic flexure becomes interposed between the right hemidiaphragm and the liver. This has been called "Chilaiditi's syndrome." A painless, gas-filled segment of colon above the dome of the right lobe of the liver may be discovered only incidentally in a chest or abdominal radiograph. However, a markedly distended hepatic flexure can cause pain in the right hypochondrium or chest.

The "splenic flexure syndrome" is more frequent, because the splenic fixture, anchored high in the left upper abdominal quadrant, is the least dependent segment of the colon and hence can serve as a natural gas trap. The flexures can become distended when there is a distal obstruction, but more often exaggerated distention results from a large volume of gas accumulating in a colon unwilling to expel it. The importance of the splenic flexure syndrome is that it can mimic disease of the chest or heart. Pain, often severe, is felt in the left hypochondrium and frequently extends into the left chest and even into the left shoulder and down the arm. This, together with pressure on the left hemidiaphragm causing a sensation of shortness of breath, convinces the patient that he or she is having a "heart attack." Clues to the contrary are that pain is neither provoked by exertion nor relieved by rest and that marked tympany can be elicited in the left hypochondrium. An upright scout film of the abdomen, if taken at the time of pain, may show a splenic flexure ballooned with gas; an electrocardiograph will show no sign of actual myocardial ischemia.

Sometimes a distinction between myocardial ischemia and a functional gastrointestinal disorder is not so easy. Indeed, the two conditions can coexist. Often, exertional angina pectoris is attended by marked anxiety, which, in turn, provokes increased air-swallowing and gaseous distention of the gut. A few such patients may seek medical attention mainly because of the gaseous distress and only incidentally recall the exertional discomfort of angina (see Chapter 13).

The pain of acute appendicitis provides a prime example of the interplay and sequence of visceral and somatic transmission of painful impulses from an evolving abdominal lesion. Every clinician knows that the initial pain of developing appendicitis is felt rather vaguely in the midabdomen, often toward the epigastrium. Only some hours later does the pain shift to become sharply localized at McBurney's point in the right lower abdominal quadrant. Knowing the difference and relation between visceral and somatic pain makes this typical sequence readily understandable. Early changes confined to the appendiceal lumen and wall stimulate nociceptors whose impulses are transmitted only along visceral pathways. The pain thus perceived is dull and referred to the midline; often it is attended by nausea. Later, as the enlarging phlegmon of the appendix touches the parietal peritoneum, parietal nociceptors are acutely stimulated. As a consequence, pain shifts, becomes sharper, and is focused at the anatomic site of the inflamed appendix. A similar sequence often occurs with acute diverticulitis affecting the sigmoid segment of colon, although, of course, the later parietal pain is felt in the left lower abdominal quadrant.

Rectal and Pelvic Pain

Rectal and pelvic pain is among the most tormenting pains related to abdominal viscera. In part, this is because the anus and rectum are richly invested with nociceptors. Thus, even a small lesion can induce severe pain. The location itself seems to lend a peculiarly uncomfortable and noisome quality to such pain which, in many cases, is not easily relieved.

Acute anorectal pain usually indicates a relatively benign condition such as mucosal fissure or fistula. Hemorrhoids alone, when confined to their origin above the pectinate line (often referred to as "internal" hemorrhoids) usually are painless, but when engorged and subject to prolapse, as so-called "external" hemorrhoids, they can be exquisitely painful. Perianal or pararectal abscess, probably because it impinges on a confined space, can also be intensely painful.

There is a fairly common, acute, remittent and recurrent rectal pain that should be readily recognized and identified by its clinical features. This is *proctalgia fugax,* aptly named a "fleeting pain in the arse." It is encountered more often in men than in women, and it has the peculiar ability to wake the victim from a sound sleep at night. In fact, it is an almost exclusively nocturnal pain. The onset of pain is usually abrupt and quite unpredictable; there is no premonitory bowel disturbance. A deep rectal ache persists for varying periods, usually about 15 minutes (although it can seem much longer to the sufferer). Probably the pain is transmitted along visceral afferent pathways, because the patient, when afflicted, typically is restless and prompted to pace the floor. The pain then recedes and disappears as spontaneously as it began. Recurring episodes vary in intensity. Symptom-free intervals range from days to months.

Rarely have patients been examined when the evanescent pain is present; either then or later no physical abnormality can be detected. A cause of proctalgia fugax has been assumed to be muscular spasm. The important point is for the clinician to be able to recognize the typical syndrome from the patient's description, thereby avoiding futile and unnecessarily involved diagnostic and therapeutic ventures.

---

*"**R**ecognizing the typical syndrome of proctalgia fugax helps avoid futile diagnostic and therapeutic ventures."*

Chronic, unrelenting pelvic pain is a common complaint and is almost always encountered in women, particularly middle-aged. Typically, the pain is described as constant, unremitting, and present day and night for weeks, months, or years without respite. Repeated examinations disclose no apparent cause, although in some instances pelvic venography may disclose vascular congestion.[13] Gynecologists are familiar with the condition and sometimes refer to it as the "pelvic floor tension syndrome." Pelvic pain in women often is aggravated by protracted standing, walking, or pushing a vacuum sweeper. Associated symptoms include dysmenorrhea, dyspareunia, and postcoital ache. Only the resolute, confident clinician can resist the temptation to perform some sort of therapeutic procedure. Usually the patient has been seen by a series of less-than-resolute physicians and tells of a series of attempted maneuvers, all to no avail. Many of these women so sadly afflicted will be found to have an attendant, often severe, mental depression. Doubtless some are depressed because of the unrelenting pain, but one can hardly avoid a suspicion that the pelvic pain may be an expression of depression.

Liver Pain

The parenchyma of the liver is relatively insensitive to pain. The capsule of the liver, on the other hand, is abundantly supplied with nociceptors. Anyone who has performed needle biopsy of the liver (or anyone who has had his or her liver biopsied) knows this. It is the penetration of the liver capsule that hurts.

In patients with liver disease, it is penetration, stretching, or distortion of Glisson's capsule that gives rise to liver pain. Depending on which lobe of the liver is mainly affected, pain typically is felt in either subcostal area; because a larger area of the liver is on the right, pain is more often in the right hypochondrium. With stimulation of adjacent parietal surfaces, pain may extend to the chest or back.

The acuity and intensity of liver pain depend a good deal on the rate at which the liver capsule has been stretched or distorted. Rapid enlargement of the liver can be acutely and intensely painful. The liver swells because something is added to its substance: fluid (including blood, by focal hemorrhage or diffuse engorgement), fat, inflammatory infiltrate, or neoplastic cells. The addition of fluid is apt to be the most abrupt, as in acute, passive hyperemia consequent to sudden right ventricular cardiac failure. I have seen patients whose mitral valve disease produced a suddenly intolerable burden on the right ventricle, whose livers became abruptly distended with congested venous blood, and whose sudden, sharp pain in the right hypochondrium at first suggested the pain of gallstone disease. Chronic right ventricular failure, as the result of longstanding pulmonary disease, results in a more gradual congestion in the liver and slower stretching of Glisson's capsule. This can produce discomfort in the right hypochondrium also, but pain is slower to appear and more of a dull ache.

Fatty metamorphosis of the liver is such a slow and gradual process that stretching of the capsule proceeds at only a snail's pace. Therefore, a fatty liver can become huge and yet be relatively painless.

The pain of diffuse inflammatory infiltrate (i.e., hepatitis) also depends on the rapidity of the inflammatory process. Acute hepatitis, with rapid swelling of the liver, often is painful; chronic hepatitis usually is not. Focal suppurative inflammation (i.e., liver abscess) is painful according to the rate at which the abscess cavity expands and the extent to which it impinges on the liver capsule. A rapidly expanding abscess near the liver surface can be acutely painful.

Neoplasia within the liver is notably painless. In part, this is because neoplasms, both primary and metastatic, typically take root and grow slowly within the parenchyma of the liver. Even neoplasms eventually encroaching on the liver surface are commonly painless, perhaps because nociceptors are destroyed in the process.

Biliary Tract Pain

When due to calculous biliary tract disease, biliary tract pain is surely among the most acute and intense pains provoked by intra-abdominal lesions. However, it is important to remember that biliary tract pain evolves in a manner similar to that described previously for appendicitis. Hypertonicity in the gallbladder or bile ducts is first registered by nociceptors served by visceral afferent pathways. Thus, the initial pain of biliary tract disease is rather vaguely centered in the epigastrium. Only when impulses become so strong as to incite activity in adjacent neurons of the dorsal spinal cord horn, or when a swollen, inflamed gallbladder triggers parietal nociceptors, does pain become sharp and localized along the right rib margin, from which it is typically referred to the right scapular area. This is why early and mild biliary tract pain—being felt in the midepigastrium rather than along the right costal margin, and being dull rather than sharp—can be symptomatically deceptive.

Some patients say that their biliary tract pain was first noted in the right hypochondrium. In most such instances, this is because the patient was awakened from sleep by pain (calculous biliary tract disease typically "acts up" in the late evening or during the night); the patient slept through the early, vague, midline pain and became aware of pain only after it had evolved to a more localized perception. In a patient whose gallbladder was previously removed, the pain of common duct stone usually is felt in the midline rather than in the right hypochondrium.

Gradual dilatation of bile ducts, as when the channel is slowly narrowed and then obstructed, by stricture or neoplasia, is often painless. For example, patients with so-called Klatskin tumors encroaching on the lumen of the common hepatic duct typically complain of jaundice first and pain later, if at all. Lesions in the porta hepatis, if they give rise to pain, tend to produce dull epigastric discomfort.

One often hears of biliary tract pain being described as "biliary colic." This is a misnomer. Biliary tract pain is not "colicky" but rather is sustained. Typically it does not come and go, but steadily rises to a peak of sharpness, maintains its painful grip with varying degrees of intensity, then eventually subsides. It is the varying intensity that may be thought to simulate colic. The distinction is that biliary tract pain does not momentarily remit and recur, as does classic colic.

"Biliary colic" is a misnomer."

Pancreatic Pain

Patients whom I have observed have convincingly demonstrated that pancreatic pain can be peculiarly disagreeable. In acute conditions, such as pancreatitis, it can become nearly unbearable. In more chronic conditions, such as carcinoma, it can be of such an onerous, oppressive character as to lead to despair.

Pancreatic pain, coming as it does from an organ buried deeply in the upper abdomen, its substance served by visceral afferent neural fibers, is usually felt in the midepigastrium. Initial impulses carried along visceral afferent pathways convey a message of pain that is somewhat vague, a deep dull ache, centered at the midline. As these visceral impulses increase in frequency and amplitude, they readily "spill over" to excite other afferent neurons in the same segment of the spinal cord, thus extending pain to either the right or left hypochondrium, depending on the preponderant focus of the noxious stimulus within the pancreas. More of the pancreas extends to the left, and the typical site of referral is to the left rib margin and flank.

Because the body of the pancreas adheres closely to the bodies of the upper lumbar vertebrae, pain from an expanding pancreatic lesion typically penetrates to the back. Pain in the posterior parietes tends to be marked by a telltale relation to posture (Figs. 2–6, 7). The patient with pancreatic pain is inclined to crouch in an attempt to ease distress; hyperextension of the back, which the patient strongly resists, tends to aggravate pancreatic pain. The patient with severe pancreatic pain typically will be found curled up in bed or bending over the edge of his or her chair or bed, with arms embracing the upper abdomen, thighs flexed against the abdomen. If the patient walks, he or she stoops.

When the lesion is acute pancreatitis and harshly irritating proteolytic juices seep from the pancreas, parietal afferent pathways are promptly invoked. If proteolytic necrosis is confined to the lesser peritoneal sac, midepigastric pain is intensified. When proteolytic irritation extends to the parietal peritoneum, pain is more sharply localized and attended by adjacent muscle guarding. Proteolytic juice seeping from an injured pancreas tends to seek egress, sometimes at considerable distances from the pancreas. It can ascend, causing pain in the chest, usually in and around the left pleural space, even into the mediastinum. It can descend along the peritoneal gutters, causing pain in the lower abdomen and pelvis. Tissue injury consequent to pancreatitis has been recorded as high as the neck and head and as low as the scrotum.

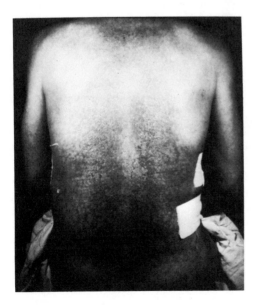

FIGURE 2–6. This 46-year-old man complained of recurring epigastric pain that was most intense where it penetrated to his back. When he stripped to the waist, the skin overlying his lumbar area was seen to be a fiery, mottled red, a sign of "erythema ab igne." His explanation was that, to relieve his back pain, he had spent much of the night huddled in a shower with scalding water pounding on his back. The diagnosis was chronic relapsing pancreatitis.

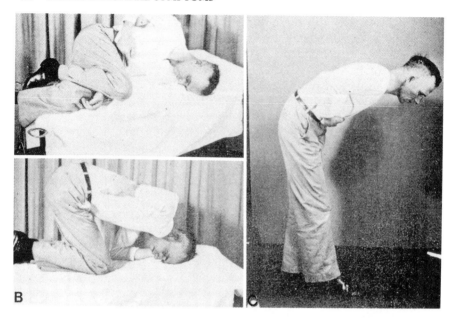

FIGURE 2-7.   Postures frequently assumed by a patient with pain arising from the pancreas or posterior parietes, as might be seen in a patient with carcinoma or a deeply penetrating peptic ulcer. A, lying curled up in a lateral decubitus position. B, knee-chest position; C, Stooping with pressure applied to the epigastrium. (Reproduced with permission from Smith LA, Rivers AB. Peptic ulcer: Pain patterns, diagnosis, and medical treatment. New York: Appleton-Century-Crofts, 1953;253.)

As a student I was taught, erroneously, that pancreatic carcinoma typically gave rise to painless jaundice. Such was the teaching in a number of schools for more than a generation of students. Nothing could be further from the truth. Pancreatic cancer in most cases is painful. Perhaps when the lesion is very small and confined within the parenchyma of the gland, pain may be dull and nondescript. But a pancreatic carcinoma of any size becomes onerously and unrelentingly painful. (Possibly the older teachers were confusing carcinoma of the common bile duct or of the papilla of Vater with carcinoma of the pancreas; the former conditions can cause painless jaundice.)

There is yet another peculiar symptomatic feature of pancreatic carcinoma. The patient so afflicted is commonly and visibly depressed. One can imagine that a patient knowing he or she harbors a pancreatic cancer might be given to despair, but even more striking is the fact that often the signs of depression precede the perception of actual pancreatic pain. It is not unusual for the patient with pancreatic cancer to have consulted specialists in various fields before the true diagnosis is established. He or she may have seen a rheumatologist or orthopaedist because of back pain; the patient may have counseled with a psychologist or psychiatrist because of his or her depression. Because an accurate diagnosis of pancreatic cancer is so often elusive, the patient's depression only deepens.

Pain Arising Within the Abdominal Wall

Occasionally, a patient will point to a place on the abdominal wall where he or she feels pain, and a suspicion arises that the inciting lesion is within the wall itself and not in underlying viscera. The patient may be able to tell the pain is superficial rather than deep. Another clue may be that the pain began and has remained in a well-localized area of the abdominal wall. Lesions within the wall tend initially to stimulate somatoparietal nociceptors; there is not a vague, diffuse, premonitory soreness typical of impulses discharged along visceral afferent pathways. Acute, focal, superficial tenderness is another sign. This can be brought out if the patient is asked to tense his or her abdomen and superficial tenderness persists; tensing the wall tends to shield the viscera, thus lessening tenderness over deep-seated lesions.

An example of an abdominal wall lesion is a muscular tear, which may also be evident by the bruised blush of an associated hematoma. Another example is an epiplocele (i.e., a herniation of preperitoneal fat) that becomes strangulated in a channel where an artery enters the rectus muscle. In this condition, typically there is exquisite tenderness of a button-like induration at a midpoint in either rectus muscle.

Somewhat more subtle is "segmental or parietal neuralgia," actually a focus of referred pain, traceable to irritation along the course of afferent nerves serving the abdominal wall. Clues to this condition include (1) aggravation of pain by movement or manipulation of the torso and by thumping over the lumbar spine and (2) hypoesthesia or hyperesthesia in the skin overlying the site. Also, the patient, if asked, often can recall paresthesias (tingling or formication) at the affected area. Two maneuvers may help to bolster a diagnosis of abdominal wall neuralgia. One is to direct a spray of ethyl chloride to the painful area; the intense cold thus produced is a counterirritant that "shuts the gate" on transmission of painful impulses. The response is immediate and sometimes surprisingly longlasting. Another is to abolish focal pain by injecting the offending superficial nerve tract with a local anesthetic agent.

Abdominal Pain Arising from Lesions That Are Not Abdominal

One must remain mindful that every instance of what the patient perceives as pain in the abdomen is not necessarily caused by an intra-abdominal lesion. For example, basilar pneumonia can cause pain beneath the costal margins, simulating hepatobiliary or pancreatic pain. Irritation anywhere along the lumbar afferent nerve tracts, from the fibers of first-order neurons, through the dorsal roots, in the dorsal horn, or along ascending paths in the spinal cord, can be registered as abdominal pain. Such irritation can occur as a result of spinal deformity, in certain forms of vertebral arthritis, in cases of perineural or paraspinal abscess, or as a result of intrinsic neuritis, such as that associated with herpes zoster infection. In such instances, the correct diagnosis becomes evident when intra-abdominal disease or injury has been excluded and when other signs of neurologic impairment, such as cutaneous anesthesia or paresthesia, can be demonstrated.

To Sum Up

The Five W's

A revealing history is compiled by a clinician in the same manner in which a newsworthy story is compiled by a journalist. Journalists are taught to include in their stories the five W's—who, what, where, when, and why. The conscientious clinician seeks to describe the first four W's in order to arrive at the why, which is an explanatory diagnosis.

Who? Who is the patient? It makes a considerable difference if the patient is an elderly person, borne down by the vicissitudes of life and keenly sensitive to pain or, in contrast, if the patient is an otherwise hale and hearty young athlete to whom a similar pain may be only a minor nuisance. Even more striking is the case of the soldier cut down by a grievous wound, yet feeling no pain because this, for him, is a "million-dollar wound," freeing him from the perils of war. Who is the patient? Is it a person who has had experience, eagerly recounted, of all sorts of pain? Or is it a person for whom pain is a new and unique happening? Who is the patient? Is it a young woman so busily engaged in her normal activity that she is distracted from her pain? Or is it a disabled elderly man who is not at all occupied except by his pain?

> *"The four 'W's—Who, What, Where, When— fashion the key to Why, the fifth 'W.' (Adapted from* The Serving Men, *by Rudyard Kipling.)"*

What? What does the patient actually feel? Is it a vague discomfort, or is it a sharply localized pain? Is it knifelike, knotlike, boring, gnawing, burning, aching? As mentioned earlier, the average patient's vocabulary is limited in describing the nuances of pain or discomfort. The inquirer cannot be satisfied with learning only that "it hurts." Usually, the patient has to be prompted and drawn out to learn what he or she really feels.

What is the patient's appearance while describing his or her symptoms? Is the reaction appropriate to the story being told? Gray and co-workers confirmed in a prospective evaluation that patients with nonspecific abdominal pain tended to close their eyes while the abdomen was being palpated.[14] There may be similar significance in the "closed-eye sign" when it is observed while the patient describes distress. And perhaps the same might be said of the patient who insists on wearing dark glasses in the subdued light of the consultation chamber.

Where? Where is the pain felt? Asking the patient to point out or to trace the site of pain is the most helpful maneuver. "Show me where it hurts" conveys not only a keen concern by the physician but enables the patient to indicate the location of pain much better than any verbal description could. Remember, too, to ask the patient if the pain started and then stayed at the place indicated or whether the pain may have started elsewhere and then shifted its locale.

When? Reconstructing the sequence of events associated with the pain, from its onset through its evolution, particularly relating the pain to what else was happening at the time, may be the most important query of all. When did the pain begin? The onset may have been so vague as to defy recall. Or the patient may be able to time the onset to a particular hour or even minute. What was the patient doing when the pain came on? Was it before or after a meal? Was it during the night? Did the pain awaken the patient, or did the patient awaken for some other reason and then become conscious of pain? In the case of recurrent pain, what seems to provoke exacerbations of pain? Occasionally one can get a helpful answer when one asks, "Not that we want you to have pain, but tell me what we might do to bring the pain on." How long did the pain last? (This is a question to which one may or may not get an accurate answer. The duration of a painful episode is sometimes exaggerated.) When does the pain ease and what, if anything, seems to relieve it? Inherent in this question is the matter of postural relief, which is seldom, if ever, volunteered and must be specifically sought. If this feature is admitted, it is helpful to ask the patient to demonstrate the relieving posture.

Why? If one can answer the pertinent questions relating to who, what, where, and when, then one has a good chance of being close to an answer of "why?", and knowing why is tantamount to having a diagnosis.

☐ *Illustrative Case*

A 62-year-old salesman called for an urgent appointment in the clinic, saying, "Last night I had a real zinger of a stomach pain." His name was immediately recognized because, even though he had never previously been registered, his wife had been a frequent visitor to the clinic, her record having accumulated in a "thick-file case." The evening before, when he was about to retire, he became aware of dull discomfort "in my stomach" (he pointed to his midepigastrium). By rapid crescendo this became an acute soreness, attended by nausea but not vomiting. Within a half-hour, pain had shifted and become sharper along the midportion of the right costal margin, from which it then extended to the right scapula. He felt feverish and then had a shaking chill. His wife insisted that he summon a physician or repair to an emergency room, but he refused. Within an hour or so the pain gradually began to ease. He had sat up most of the night, eventually dozing off to sleep. On awakening he felt only soreness in the right upper quadrant of his abdomen.

The patient claimed to have enjoyed good health previously. On further questioning, he recalled having had one or two similar but much less intense episodes within the preceding year. In each instance, the bout of pain lasted only a few hours, and the intervals between bouts were symptom-free. He had observed no change in his regular bowel habits or in the appearance of his urine.

Physical examination was unrevealing except for a heavy-set habitus and slight tenderness beneath the right costal margin. His temperature was normal. By the time of his morning appointment in the clinic he was fully ambulatory and relatively pain-free.

He was informed that, in addition to urinalysis, blood counts, and blood chemistry panel (all of which were normal), upper abdominal ultrasonography would be arranged later that day. As expected, this clearly showed a clump of dense concrements in the gallbladder. The liver, bile ducts, and pancreas were normal.

The patient was told that cholecystectomy was in order. I then described the operation in detail, including its minimal risks and the expected duration of hospitalization. We continued:

Physician: Do you have any questions?
Patient: Just one.
Physician: What is that?
Patient: What am I going to tell my wife?
Physician: Just what we have told you.
Patient: I don't think that will do.
Physician: Why not?
Patient: I can tell you now that she'll be upset. She'll ask, "How is it that you go to the clinic, and right away they tell you what's wrong and how to cure it? Here I've been going to the same clinic for twenty years, and no one has yet found out what's wrong with me."

I had no satisfying answer to the man's question.

Comment. This patient provided a succinct, clear-cut account of recent pain that was almost a classic textbook picture of biliary tract pain and was in sharp contrast to his wife's longstanding, nondescript complaints of abdominal distress. Little wonder that the man's narrative led to a swift resolution of his problem, whereas his poor wife was still floundering in uncertainty.

The patient's report of dull pain beginning in the midepigastrium, and then becoming more precisely localized in the right upper abdominal quadrant with extension to the right scapular area, pointed strongly to a diagnosis of calculous biliary tract disease. A minimum of investigation was required for confirmation.

To the basic tests that were ordered, I could have added determination of serum amylase and lipase activity, but there were no features suggesting an associated pancreatitis. I could also have requested barium meal radiography or have scheduled upper gastrointestinal endoscopy, but again the symptoms were not those of esophageal, gastric, or duodenal lesions. The likelihood of an upper alimentary tract survey turning up an unexpected or incidental finding of importance in the absence of suggestive symptoms is almost nil. Radiographic or endoscopic survey of the colon would have been quite beside the point of the patient's problem, although it could, perhaps, be thought of as a screening procedure.

To justify a protracted series of preoperative tests, often the argument is "The surgeon needs all the advance information he can get." Perhaps the argument should rather be phrased as "The surgeon benefits from all the information he can use." One is reminded that a well-trained, experienced surgeon is capable of deriving at the operating table a good deal of information by which to decide the procedure. In many instances, it is not necessary to prolong preoperative investigation simply to suggest to the surgeon before-hand what he or she is quite able to find out for himself or herself.

We settled, then, on the most direct approach. Cholecystectomy was performed, and the patient's convalescence was without event. He remained well. His wife remained dismayed.

References

1. Boston Med Surg J 1858; May 6.
*2. Wall PD. On the relation of injury to pain. Pain 1979; 6:253–264.
*3. Bockus HL. Abdominal pain. In: Berk JE, Haubrich WS, Kalser MH, Roth JLA, Schaffner F, eds. Bockus Gastroenterology, 4th ed. Philadelphia: WB Saunders, 1985.
4. Melzack R, Wall PD. Pain mechanisms, a new theory. Science 1965; 150:971–979.
5. Levitt RE. Newer developments in the physiology and management of abdominal pain. In: Berk JE, Haubrich WS, Kalser MH, Roth JLA, Schaffner F, eds. Bockus Gastroenterology, 4th ed. Philadelphia, WB Saunders, 1985.
*6. Engel GL. Psychogenic pain and the pain-prone patient. Am J Med 1959; 26:899–918.
7. Welgan P, Meshkinpour H, Beeler M. Effect of anger on colon motor and myoelectric activity. Gastroenterology 1988; 94:1150–1156.
8. Sherrington CS. Postural activity of muscle and nerve. Brain 1915; 38:191.
*9. Blumer D, Heilbronn M. Chronic pain as a variant of depressive disease; the pain-prone disorder. J Nerv Ment Dis 1982; 170:381–406.

*References 2, 3, 6, and 9 are worthy of more general review.

10. Minors DS, Waterhouse JM. In: Circadian rhythms and the human. Bristol: John Wright & Sons, 1981:187–244.

11. Roberts-Thomson IC, Knight RE, Kennaway DJ, Pannall PR. Circadian rhythms in patients with abdominal pain syndromes. Austr NZ J Med 1988; 18:569–574.

12. Whitehead WE, Schuster MM, Cheskin LJ, Heller BR. Exacerbation of irritable bowel syndrome during menses. [Abstract.] Gastroenterology 1988; 94:A495.

13. Beard RW, Reginald PW, Wadsworth J. Clinical features of women with chronic lower abdominal pain and pelvic congestion. Br J Obstet Gynaecol 1988; 95:153–161.

14. Gray DW, Dixon JM, Collin J. The closed eyes sign: An aid to diagnosing nonspecific abdominal pain. Br Med J 1988; 297:837.

HEARTBURN

Walter J. Hogan, M.D.

3

Definition

Heartburn is the symptom most readily identified with the gastrointestinal tract. Sometimes called "pyrosis" (from the Greek *pyr* for fire), heartburn has been defined as a "burning, tight sensation in the region of the xiphisternum, radiating upward to the neck."[1] In its classic expression, heartburn translates the distress associated with gastrointestinal reflux into a recognizable complaint.

Most of us periodically experience heartburn without apparent sequelae. However, persistent or incapacitating heartburn often signals the development of mucosal inflammation or complications arising from gastroesophageal reflux disease (GERD). Although classic heartburn implies gastroesophageal reflux, this symptom is often absent or uninterpretable in GERD, thus depriving both the patient and the clinician of a valuable, albeit discomforting, clinical warning.

Exposition of Symptoms

Geography and vector are the key features that identify classic heartburn. The burning sensation originates beneath the lower sternum (not epigastrium) and invariably rises in an orad direction, often to the level of the suprasternal notch. Heartburn may radiate to the upper back, neck, jaws, teeth, or arms, but it requires a retrosternal origin to validate its identity.[2] Not unexpectedly, the term "heartburn" is used inappropriately by many patients in attempts to describe their dyspeptic complaints. Unfortunately, physicians readily accept this complaint on faith without attempting to qualify the heartburn and to obtain a description in detail of what the patient experiences. The point to be emphasized is that one should never accept the symptom of heartburn until it has been fully described by the patient.

"The term 'heartburn' is used inappropriately by many patients."

When a dyspeptic patient is requested to trace the topography of heartburn, invariably the epigastrium or left breast is identified, and the midchest component is absent. This is *not* classic heartburn and does *not* imply the presence of gastroesophageal reflux.[3]

Acid regurgitation often accompanies the symptoms of heartburn. Patients readily complain of a "sour, bitter taste" associated with some episodes of heartburn, particularly those that awaken them from sleep. The latter may be associated with aspiration-like symptoms in severe GERD. Acid regurgitation frequently also occurs with a belch–heartburn sequence.[4]

"Water brash" sometimes accompanies the symptom of heartburn and, occasionally, may be the patient's major complaint. Water brash is the sudden increase in volume of saliva occurring as a result of reflex stimulation of the salivary glands by the same sensory receptors within the esophagus involved with the sensation described as heartburn. The patient experiences profuse salivation that may be construed incorrectly as nausea.

Pathophysiologic Mechanisms

Heartburn is caused by direct exposure of the esophageal mucosal lining to refluxed gastric contents. Although GERD is a multifactorial disorder, incompetence of the lower esophageal sphincter (LES) mechanism is the final common pathway. Gastroesophageal reflux events have been observed during concurrent monitoring of LES dynamics and intraluminal esophageal pH. These observations have identified three types of LES pressure profiles associated with gastroesophageal reflux.[5]

Transient LES relaxation has been described with spontaneous gastroesophageal reflux (Fig. 3–1). Abrupt LES relaxation occurs following periods of demonstrably normal or elevated resting LES tone (Fig. 3–1A). Transient LES relaxation is the primary phenomenon associated with gastroesophageal reflux events in normal subjects. When resting LES tone is low, rises in intraabdominal pressure cause stress-related gastroesophageal reflux. Undoubtedly this is the mechanism responsible for reflux when the patient bends, strains, or squats. Free reflux episodes can also be demonstrated during periods of low LES tone (hypotonia) without associated increases in intragastric pressure or intraluminal esophageal contractile activity (Fig. 3–1B). Although the last two mechanisms for gastroesophageal reflux are often seen, the predominant mechanism involves transient LES relaxation.

The mechanism of transient LES relaxation has yet to be defined. Most authorities believe that this alteration is mediated by the same vagal inhibitory efferent nerves associated with normal LES relaxation following swallowing. Gastric distention in humans increases the frequency of LES relaxation, and stimulation of the vagus nerve or the posterior pharynx results in similar findings in laboratory animals. Recent studies add another element in their suggestion that the mechanism(s) of transient LES relaxation may be a variant of the belch reflex.

Interestingly, although practically everyone experiences gastroesophageal reflux during a 24-hour period, the majority of reflux episodes are without symptoms.[6] Macroscopic alteration of the esophageal mucosal lining does not have to be present in association with the symptom of heartburn. In point of fact, heartburn is very common during the third trimester of pregnancy, whereas the esophagus is unscathed. Conversely, overt esophagitis is not always associated with the symptom of heartburn.[7] Nonetheless, most patients with esophagitis have heartburn as their predominant symptom, and heartburn is the primary reason for their seeking medical advice.

"The majority of reflux episodes are without symptoms."

The process by which heartburn is perceived is unknown. Afferent nerve receptors in the esophagus apparently transmit the message concerning gastroesophageal reflux to the brain, but the definitive exciting mechanism has not been elucidated. As noted earlier, heartburn is associated with a predictable, significant increase in saliva production;[8] however, even though there is gastroesophageal reflux, salivary flow does not increase if the symptom of heartburn is not experienced.[9] This observation suggests that the neuronal receptors that cause heartburn also stimulate salivary flow—an obvious at-

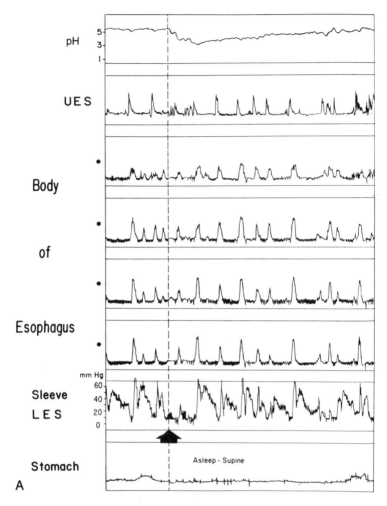

FIGURE 3-1. A, Esophageal manometric tracing demonstrating transient relaxation of the lower esophageal sphincter (LES) immediately following a period of elevated LES pressure in a patient who is asleep (*arrow*). A drop in intraluminal esophageal pH is noted at the top of the tracing. Concomitant contractile events in the upper esophageal sphincter (UES), the body of the esophagus, and the stomach are also recorded. LES pressure was continuously monitored using a Dent sleeve sensor. B, Esophageal manometric tracing demonstrating gastroesophageal reflux (pH recording at top) during a prolonged period of low LES pressure (hypotonia) (*arrow*).

tempt to enhance esophageal acid clearance and relieve the burning distress. Along similar lines, heartburn is less frequent in patients with peptic stricture formation. Is the symptom of heartburn, therefore, an integral part of an esophageal protective mechanism against the potential ravages of gastric contents?

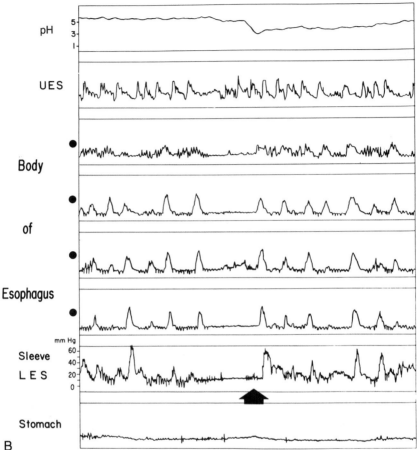

FIGURE 3-1. *B Continued*

Clinical Features

Identification of classic heartburn depends on the presence of five key clinical features: (1) characterization of the distress; (2) origination; (3) radiation; (4) precipitating events; and (5) relief pattern (Table 3-1).

Heartburn characteristically burns or sears and a sense of pressure or tightening of the chest may accompany the burning. The burning originates beneath the xiphisternum and radiates upward beneath the sternum. The orad component is almost always present, although it may extend for only a few centimeters. The burning sensation can radiate to the upper neck, jaws, shoulders, or arms and, when severe erosive esophagitis is present, may travel into

TABLE 3–1. Key Clinical Features of Classic Heartburn

- Characterization of distress
- Origination
- Radiation
- Precipitating events
- Relief pattern

the upper midback.[10] Heartburn is typically provoked by eating and by lying down; it often occurs shortly after retiring at nighttime, especially if the patient has eaten immediately before retiring.

Uncomplicated heartburn predictably dissipates within a few minutes following antacid ingestion, but symptoms may recur within a short time. Because heartburn recurs so soon, patients frequently deny experiencing relief with antacids because the respite was temporary; if this sequence is pointed out to them, they often revise their story. When severe erosive esophagitis is present, however, relief of heartburn with antacids is often ineffective compared with earlier stages of the disease. Once again, this alteration in antacid efficacy needs to be revealed by careful questioning of the patient. It helps to ask if and how the symptom has changed since its onset.

Significance Within Clinical Setting

Both heartburn and acid regurgitation are considered to be very sensitive and specific symptoms for GERD. This is particularly the case if these symptoms are provoked by food intake, recumbency, or stooping. Unfortunately, it has been demonstrated repeatedly since the advent of ambulatory esophageal pH monitoring that only a minority of gastroesophageal reflux episodes are perceived symptomatically by patients. This is true even in those who actually experience heartburn at sometime during the pH recording. Additionally, other nonspecific symptoms have been associated with gastroesophageal reflux, including nausea, belching, epigastric pain, retrosternal (nonradiating) pain or burning, and chest pain. How significant, therefore, are symptoms relative to GERD, particularly heartburn and acid regurgitation?

In a recent report, symptoms of gastroesophageal reflux were evaluated in a group of 304 patients referred for 24-hour esophageal pH monitoring. Previous to pH monitoring, each patient was interviewed by an experienced gastroenterologist. The patient described his or her symptoms and then completed a standard symptom questionnaire. Thereupon, the physician was asked to make two determinations: (1) to judge whether the patient had gastroesophageal reflux based on the subjective information, and (2) to decide whether one symptom clearly dominated among the complaints.

Heartburn and acid regurgitation were the only symptoms differing significantly in frequency between groups of patients with normal and abnormal pH monitoring studies. However, nearly half of the patients with normal pH monitoring also reported these two symptoms. Nonetheless, when heartburn or acid regurgitation were the predominant symptoms, they had a high specificity (89 percent and 95 percent, respectively) but a low sensitivity (38 percent and 6 percent, respectively) for GERD. No preliminary diagnosis could be rendered concerning the presence or absence of GERD in a third of the patient group because of "inconclusive symptomatology" at the time of history review.

Two possible reasons were advanced to explain why a substantial proportion of patients with GERD have nonspecific symptoms. First, when the patient and physician discuss a symptom such as heartburn, the term used to denote the symptom may not mean the same thing to the patient and the physician. Second, ill-defined feelings may be expressed, just as they commonly are in other disorders in which initial symptoms are transmitted along visceral neural pathways (see Chapter 2, "Abdominal Pain").

> *"Heartburn' may not mean the same thing to the patient and the physician."*

Two important points were established by this study:

1. Predominant complaints of heartburn or acid regurgitation are "typical" and specific for GERD.
2. When these symptoms are absent, the presence of GERD cannot be excluded.

Diagnosis

Differential Diagnosis

Retrosternal "burning" may occur with a variety of clinical conditions involving several organ systems, including the heart, gallbladder, stomach, duodenum, and colon. The difficulty in distinguishing pain of esophageal origin from angina pectoris is legendary. This type of retrosternal distress does not possess the key features of classic heartburn, however, and a careful history should help exclude GERD.[11] An important point to be made concerns heartburn in patients with esophageal motor disorders, particularly achalasia.[12] The patient with esophageal dysmotility describes retrosternal burning that many times is relieved by water, carbonated drinks, or antacids; it has no orad radiation. In these patients, investigation discloses no mucosal inflammation as seen with GERD. This type of burning is apparently caused by esophageal spasm or by fermentation of retained food, because it tends to improve following brusque (pneumatic) dilatation of the esophageal narrowing.

Heartburn is a common complaint of women during the third trimester of pregnancy. This phenomenon may provide an advantage to the physician investigating the nature of heartburn in a woman. Misunderstanding the symptoms of heartburn seldom exists when a woman has previously experienced "heartburn of pregnancy." Needless to say, the patient usually has to be asked by the physician examiner to recall this experience.

A substantial body of information and recorded observations exists concerning certain food substances and their potential to cause heartburn. Fatty foods, alcohol, chocolate, and spicy foods, which usually head the list of offending substances, apparently influence resting LES tone.[13] The patient usually recalls specific foods that precipitate heartburn, but it may be difficult for the physician to decide whether it is the content or the bulk of the meal that is the offending factor. This feature of the history adds little weight to the authenticity of the complaint of heartburn since "food intolerance" is a common complaint of the dyspeptic patient.[14]

An interesting variation of heartburn may occur in the patient with an extensive columnar-lined (Barrett's) esophagus or peptic stricture formation— both complications of longstanding GERD. Early on there may have been frequent episodes of heartburn, prompting antacid ingestion extending for years or even decades. Later, heartburn gradually dissipates and may have disappeared by the time medical attention is sought. This seeming improvement belies the complications of GERD; the columnar-type epithelium may not provide the sensory mechanism necessary to translate reflux into heartburn, or stricture may deny access of gastric contents into the esophagus. Dysphagia may be the trade-off symptom in this evolutionary process and it is difficulty in swallowing that eventually prompts the patient to seek medical advice.

Distinction Between Regurgitation and Vomiting

Regurgitation, a phenomenon most often associated with gastroesophageal reflux conditions, is the relatively effortless upheaval of fluid or food into the esophagus that frequently occurs with a "belch," or increased pressure transient (gradient) within the stomach. For gastroesophageal reflux or regurgitation to occur, LES pressure must be reduced to the equivalent of intragastric pressure. Such transient LES relaxations are more frequent with increased intragastric pressure caused by air insufflation and possibly by meals. The belch mechanism may be very similar to that of acid reflux (see Chapter 12, "Gaseousness") for, not uncommonly, acid reflux is evident at the same time that a "belch event" is signaled by the patient during a 24-hour esophageal intraluminal pH study.

The often sizable amounts of fluid and/or food regurgitated into the esophagus during an episode of LES relaxation may ascend to the upper esophagus.

Frequently associated with the delivery of these substances to this level is a sour taste, burning, or aspiration-like symptoms, depending on the volume of the gastric contents and the posture of the patient.

It should be pointed out that regurgitation may be a learned response in some situations. Merycism, for example, is a childhood form of "pleasurable" regurgitation whereby the regurgitated bolus is chewed and reswallowed, and the process continued until the food empties into the duodenum (see Chapter 14, "Eating Disorders").

In contrast to regurgitation, vomiting is the forceful expulsion of gastric contents (see Chapter 5, "Nausea and Vomiting"). Unlike regurgitation, vomiting is associated with nausea and water brash. It also is attended by retching or straining as part of a complex interaction of proximal duodenal/gastric and abdominal wall contractions with receptive relaxation of the diaphragm. Vomiting seldom is associated with ordinary GERD and, in general, is rare in most instances of complicated reflux disease.

*"**R**egurgitation, in contrast to vomiting, is not associated with nausea or attended by retching."*

Diagnostic Studies

The symptom of heartburn generally does not require extensive diagnostic study if it is self-limited and controlled by conservative measures or short-term medication. It is impossible to decide from the symptom alone whether heartburn signifies submucosal inflammatory alteration, but this is a moot point if the heartburn is temporary and responsive. If the heartburn becomes persistent or aggressive, however, an inflamed esophageal lining probably exists and diagnostic work-up is indicated. If dysphagia occurs with heartburn, immediate investigation is mandated.

The barium-contrast esophagogram remains the first-line study to evaluate dysphagia and possible peptic stricture formation. Unfortunately, the esophagogram—even when employing a double-contrast technique—remains a relatively insensitive test to detect inflammatory changes of esophagitis (Fig. 3-2). An esophagogastroduodenal endoscopic examination with tissue biopsy is the diagnostic procedure of choice to substantiate the presence of esophagitis and its complications, such as Barrett's columnar-lined esophagus.

Ambulatory 24-hour pH recording is a useful test to establish gastroesopha-

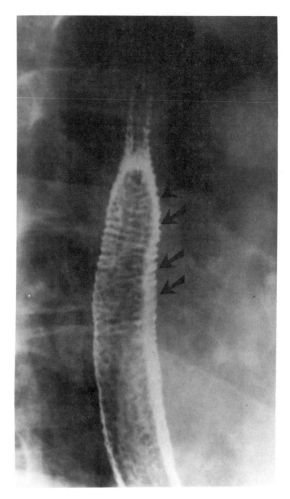

FIGURE 3-2. Although the double-contrast esophagogram often cannot define mucosal changes associated with gastroesophageal reflux, this was not the situation with this heartburn sufferer. The air–barium coating in this esophagogram clearly identifies the mucosal serrations (*arrows*) associated with peptic esophagitis. This is an example of "felinization," an inflammatory condition in humans that simulates the appearance of the cat esophagus.

geal reflux and the possible association of heartburn with demonstrable reflux events. The test is most useful in detecting subtle GERD in certain clinical conditions, such as noncardiac chest pain.[15] However, in the presence of classic heartburn and demonstrated mucosal inflammation, an ambulatory pH study adds little additional information.

Illustrative Case

A 26-year-old technical student presents with a chief complaint of persistent "heartburn." He describes this as episodic, low substernal burning that occurs after meals and frequently awakens him from sleep. Upon a request to indicate the location of the heartburn with his finger, the patient traced a pathway from the subxiphoid up to the midsternum.

The symptom is longstanding, having been noted recurrently over the past decade. At times it has been intense but controllable with antacid tablets. On occasion, the patient consumed a whole roll of Tums in a single day!

The heartburn became intensified during the last 6 months of school, especially during examinations. The substernal burning now is no longer responsive to antacids and, because of this, the patient has been losing sleep. The distress is aggravated by tomato-based sauces, fried onions, pizza, chocolate, and red wine. Recently, the patient has become aware of heartburn while jogging. Both heartburn and regurgitation of sour-tasting juice occur sometimes when he is bending over to "work on the car motor."

There is no pain from or difficulty in swallowing. The patient's father is said to have self-treated a similar condition for many years.

Endoscopy disclosed extensive distal esophagitis involving the lower 6 centimeters of the esophagus with linear, confluent erosions throughout the circumference. A relatively large, sliding hiatus hernia was also present. There was no wall compliance in the distal esophagus with insufflated air.

Symptoms virtually disappeared when omeprazole was given for 8 weeks but recurred almost immediately following discontinuation of the drug. Omeprazole therapy was reinstituted, and once again the symptoms were relieved. A fundoplication operation was discussed, but the patient was reticent to undergo a major operation.

Comment. This case emphasizes the chronicity of heartburn and the preservation of its characteristics despite years of occurrence. The heartburn and gastroesophageal reflux have waxed and waned over the years but, for the most part, had been "controlled" by self-medication with antacids. (I suspect this is not an unusual story and typifies the majority of heartburn sufferers.) However, the heartburn was no longer responsive, the sleeping pattern had been disturbed, and medical help was now sought. There is no odynophagia or dysphagia that would signal a more aggressive chapter in the scenario of GERD. The intensity and longevity of the symptoms in such a young man provokes concern, and the apparent association of heightened sensitivity with school examinations is noteworthy.

The symptoms were readily controlled with omeprazole, although larger doses were necessary (20 mg twice daily) during periods of examination stress. The free regurgitation and postural aggravation of symptoms disappeared as long as the medication was maintained. However, the long history of GERD, the relatively refractive esophagitis, and the nature of this chronic recurrent disease mandate the need for continuous potent medication or, more than likely, eventual surgical intervention.

To Sum Up

Heartburn and acid regurgitation are sensitive indicators of GERD. Unfortunately, these symptoms are not sensitive in detecting GERD. A careful review of the key features associated with the symptom of heartburn should help the physician to differentiate classic heartburn from other types of chest and retrosternal distress in most instances. An essential element in this differentiation is derived from the patient's own description and characterization of his or her heartburn. To secure all the details calls for good listening and communication skills by the interviewing physician, which, after all, are the basic requisites for obtaining an accurate and informative medical history.

References

1. Fleming PR. Heartburn. In: Hart FD, ed. French's index of differential diagnosis. 12th ed. Bristol: Wright, 1985:378.
2. Klauser AG, Schindlbeck NE, Müeller-Lissner SA. Symptoms in gastro-oesophageal reflux disease. Lancet 1990; 335:205–208.
3. Horrocks JC, DeDombal FT. Clinical presentation of patients with "dyspepsia." Detailed symptomatic study of 360 patients. Gut 1978; 19:19–26.
4. Hope RA, Longmore JM, Moss PAH, Warrens AN. Oxford handbook of clinical medicine. 2nd ed. Oxford: Oxford University Press, 1989:22.
5. Hogan WJ, Dodds WJ. Gastroesophageal reflux disease. In: Sleisenger MH, Fordtran JS, eds. Gastrointestinal disease. 4th ed. Philadelphia: WB Saunders, 1989:594–619.
6. Fuchs KH, DeMeester TR, Albertucci M. Specificity and sensitivity of objective diagnosis of gastroesophageal reflux disease. Surgery 1987; 102:575–580.
7. Smith JL, Opekun AR, Larkai E, Graham DY. Sensitivity of the esophageal mucosa to pH in gastroesophageal reflux disease. Gastroenterology 1989; 96:683–689.
8. Helm JF, Dodds WJ, Hogan WJ. Salivary response to esophageal acid in normal subjects and patient with reflux esophagitis. Gastroenterology 1987; 93:1393–1397.
9. Helm JF, Allendorph M, Dodds WJ, et al. Loss of the salivary response to esophageal acid perfusion in patients with peptic stricture. Gastroenterology, 1986; 90(5):1456.
10. Johnson F, Joelsson B, Gudmundsson K, Greiff L. Symptoms and endoscopic findings in the diagnosis of gastroesophageal reflux disease. Scand J Gastroenterol 1987; 22:714–718.
11. Davies HA, Jones DB, Rhodes J, Newcombe RG. Angina-like esophageal pain: Differentiation from cardiac pain by history. J Clin Gastroenterol 1985; 7:477–481.
12. Smart HL, Foster PN, Evans DF, et al. Twenty-four hour oesophageal acidity in achalasia before and after pneumatic dilatation. Gut 1987; 28:883–887.
13. Richter JE, Castell DO. Gastroesophageal reflux: Pathogenesis, diagnosis, and therapy. Ann Intern Med 1982; 97:93–103.
14. Horrocks JC, De Dombal FT. Diagnosis of dyspepsia from data collected by a physician's assistant. Br Med J 1975; 3:421–423.
15. Klauser AG, Heinrich C, Schindelbeck NE, Müeller-Lissner SA. Is long-term esophageal pH monitoring of clinical value? Am J Gastroenterol 1989; 84:362–366.

SWALLOWING PROBLEMS: DYSPHAGIA AND ODYNOPHAGIA

Walter J. Hogan, M.D.

4

Difficulty experienced during the act of swallowing food or water is termed "dysphagia," a term derived from the Greek word meaning "difficulty in eating." Dysphagia, one of the few specific target symptoms related to the gastrointestinal tract, implies a significant problem with esophageal structure or function. Encompassed in the term dysphagia is a spectrum of sensations ranging from a temporary "hang-up" of food following ingestion to total obstruction of the transit of food or fluid through the esophagus. Painful swallowing, a distinct sensation that stands apart from dysphagia, is called "odynophagia." Although this term often is applied to a condition associated with bacterial or viral pharyngitis, it principally refers to esophageal pain occurring during transport of food or liquid through the gullet.

Dysphagia can involve two major anatomic zones: (1) the oropharynx, which includes that portion of the swallowing mechanism located above the upper esophageal sphincter; and (2) the body of the esophagus, extending from the upper esophageal sphincter through the zone of the lower esophageal sphincter. Dysphagia generally occurs in the absence of odynophagia; conversely, odynophagia is almost always associated with some form of dysphagia.

Oropharyngeal Dysphagia

Illustrative Case

The patient is a 45-year-old tubing mill worker. Three months before being referred to our clinic, he developed a "sore throat." The problem persisted for a month without notable dysphagia or symptoms of reflux. Two months before being evaluated, the patient "almost choked" on a meal of crackers and cheese. Subsequently, he began to have progressive problems with solid foods. These took the form initially of "gagging and choking" and progressed to a situation in which he found himself "forever trying to get things down my throat." Ultimately this led to the complaint that "things just won't go down." Swallowing liquids posed no problem, and there were no symptoms of aspiration or pharyngeal regurgitation. Interestingly, the patient found that eventually he was unable to suck liquids through a straw. Additionally, he remarked that he seemed to have "more saliva" than previously noted, but he was not bothered by this during the night.

"A clue: he could no longer suck liquids through a straw"

His speech had become somewhat garbled, and his enunciation was impaired. His wife remarked, "He always sounds juicy now." The patient's weight had declined by at least 25 pounds in the preceding 2 months; he denied having muscle weakness, increased fatigue, arthralgia, or difficulty in swallowing pills.

Several dilations of the esophagus with large-diameter bougies had been of no avail. Radiographic examination of the esophagus by means of a barium swallow, esophagogastroscopy, examination by a laryngologist, and a complete laboratory screen were all unrevealing. The problem was not helped with medication, including H_2 receptor antagonists, nifedipine, metoclopramide, and antacids. The patient's throat had been cultured repeatedly, but no significant pathogens were detected. A standard esophageal manometric study was reported as unremarkable. A Bernstein test was negative.

Following a review of the patient's history, a "swallowing study" was recorded by videoradiography in order to observe the patient's swallowing mechanism. He could not retain a bolus of barium within his mouth, repeatedly allowing it to slip posteriorly into the hypopharynx. There was no aspiration of the barium, but he was unable to oppose the soft tissue adjacent to the base of the tongue against the posterior wall. Time and again he would lose the bolus from his mouth. He also could not suck barium through a straw.

Neurologic consultation and a computed tomography (CT) scan of the head confirmed the presence of a brain lesion, which was subsequently determined to be the result of vascular injury. Later it was learned that the patient's mother had her first "stroke" at age 61 and subsequently had difficulty speaking and swallowing; there was otherwise no familial history of similar swallowing problems.

Esophageal Dysphagia

Esophageal dysphagia may occur because of a primary functional (motor) disorder or because of an anatomic or structural alteration of the esophagus.

Primary Motor Disorder

☐ *Illustrative Case*

The patient is a 65-year-old white woman with a 4-year history of intermittent dysphagia for solids and liquids. During this period she had at least two episodes of apparently completely obstructive dysphagia. A recent work-up, including at least one esophagogastroscopy and two barium meal examinations, was essentially unremarkable except that the second radiographic examination suggested the possibility of "a distal esophageal narrowing." Bougienage dilation of the esophagus, however, did not allay the symptoms.

The patient complains that she is obliged to take considerable time eating and "never goes out" because of this handicap. She has to ingest water with each swallow and sometimes finds herself standing up, hyperextending her head, or holding her hands over her head in order to swallow. She is aware of occasional retrosternal "gurgling" and is quite astute in perceiving "when things leave my chest and go into my stomach." She complains of excessive saliva and "choking on phlegm" at times. She also describes occasional episodes of nocturnal coughing and choking. Her spouse indicates that on some occasions she awakens during the night, sits on the edge of the bed with her legs dangling over the side, and makes a noise "like a draining sink." Eventually she lies down and sleeps without further difficulty. The patient also had a history of intermittent "burning" that is relieved by Alka-Seltzer or carbonated beverages. She has not been able to belch as "fully" as she could in the past. Despite the difficulty with eating, her weight has fluctuated by only a few pounds.

"She knew 'when things leave my chest and go into my stomach.'"

Esophageal manometric study disclosed an absence of primary peristalsis within the esophagus, elevated intraluminal esophageal pressure, and ineffective relaxation of an elevated lower esophageal sphincter tone. Provocative challenge with a bolus of cholecystokinin resulted in brief, sustained contraction of the lower esophageal sphincter. A subsequent radiograph confirmed that there was no lumen-obliterating "stripping wave" below the aortic notch.

The esophagus was capable of supporting a column of barium to the level of the aortic notch without emptying. There was a typical "birdbeak" appearance to the distal esophagus at the cardioesophageal junction. Esophageal emptying was markedly enhanced when amyl nitrite was inhaled during fluoroscopic examination.

Subsequent endoscopic examination showed a closed, easily effaced esophagogastric junction that was pliable and symmetric. No lesion was evident within the zone of the cardioesophageal junction. Residual food and fluid debris had collected within a patulous, hypomotile esophagus. Numerous purposeless contractile waves were observed within the wall of the esophagus. Once or twice there was a lumen-obliterating contraction, but this appeared to be segmental and nonperistaltic.

The clinical, manometric, radiographic, and endoscopic findings were considered to be compatible with the diagnosis of esophageal achalasia.

Structural Abnormality

Illustrative Case

A 35-year-old man was referred following his second episode of obstructive dysphagia. Twice, at a hospital emergency room, an impacted food bolus had had to be removed from his distal esophagus. A recent barium-contrast esophagogram as well as an esophagogastroscopy had failed to disclose any active inflammation or detectable structural alteration of the esophagus. A hiatus hernia had been seen on both examinations, but no evidence of gastroesophageal reflux disease was apparent. The patient had a history of intermittent "heartburn" and had taken Tums intermittently for years. He claimed that he usually had little problem with eating, but the two occasions when he was obliged to seek relief in the emergency room were both preceded by eating beef at a restaurant. On further questioning, he admitted to occasional difficulty in swallowing and said that once in a while he had a brief feeling that swallowed food was "hung up" in his esophagus. There was no history of nocturnal cough or aspiration, chest trauma, or symptoms suggesting problems in the mouth or pharynx.

An esophagogram was performed during which the patient was asked to swallow a barium-impregnated marshmallow. Transit of the marshmallow was observed from the mouth into the stomach. He was able to ingest only half of the marshmallow; this was transported unimpeded to the distal esophagus where it became impacted and remained for several minutes (Fig. 4–1). Coincidentally, the patient developed symptoms similar to those that he had experienced when bits of beef had become impacted. With continued intake of barium, the marshmallow was eventually swept into the stomach and the patient felt relieved. A hiatus hernia was evident at fluoroscopy. There was one episode of barium reflux into the esophagus, which reached the level of the aortic arch. Esophagogastroscopy was repeated. This disclosed a subtle,

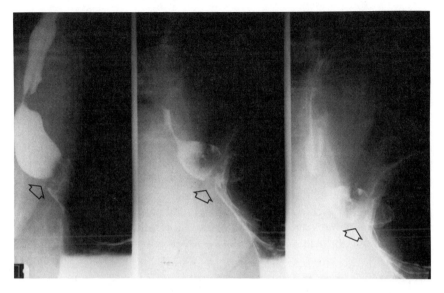

FIGURE 4-1.   Series of radiographs showing obstruction of a marshmallow to passage through a distal esophageal area of noncompliance (*arrows*). The bolus was impacted for 2$^{1}/_{2}$ to 3 minutes, during which time the patient's dysphagic symptoms were reproduced.

ringlike cicatrix at the cardioesophageal junction with "pitting" of the proximal 2 centimeters of mucosa. Several superficial erosions were noted in this segment. These findings were considered evidence of chronic reflux esophagitis with subsequent mild stricture formation and noncompliance at the distal esophagus.

Following esophageal dilation with a No. 56 French bougie, the patient remained symptom-free for 14 months. He remarked, "I am eating normally for the first time that I can remember."

> "*He thought he had little trouble swallowing,*
> *but he couldn't swallow a marshmallow.*"

Odynophagia

Illustrative Case

A 25-year-old medical student, was seen following the acute onset of "painful swallowing." This had developed 2 days before, following a "flu-like" prodrome of myalgia, sore throat, and headache. Odynophagia became so severe that the patient was unable to swallow food or fluid, including oral pain medication. At this point it seemed too painful even to swallow saliva.

Barium-contrast radiography showed relatively normal esophageal motor function but the mucosal contour was irregular throughout the lower half of the esophagus. There was no hiatus hernia and no evidence of gastroesophageal reflux. Esophagogastroscopy showed marked alterations of the esophageal mucosa with discrete, superficial, punched-out ulcerations beginning 23 cm from the incisor teeth and separated by apparently normal, uninvolved mucosa. The ulcerations became confluent at the midesophagus, and the entire distal esophagus appeared to be eroded, friable, and erythematous. Multiple mucosal biopsy specimens were obtained. Microscopic examination disclosed viral inclusion bodies typical of herpetic infection of the esophagus.

The patient was treated with intravenous fluids, parenteral pain medication, and acyclovir. Within 2 days he was able to swallow fluids, and within 5 days he could swallow normally.

Physiology and Pathophysiology Correlated with Clinical Features

Oropharyngeal swallowing events are under the exclusive control of the central nervous system.[1] This action begins at the tip of the tongue and ends when the bolus is transported to the level of the upper esophageal sphincter. The major focus of supraesophageal swallowing is to direct a bolus in such a manner as to efface a relaxed upper esophageal sphincter and to strip luminal contents efficiently from the oropharynx. Swallowing events in the oropharynx are rapid, the sequence requiring only about 1 second.

The oropharyngeal swallowing mechanism is under the control of the swallowing center in the brain stem and is also governed by cranial nerves V, VII, IX, X, and XII. Disruption of the midbrain swallowing center or any of the involved cranial nerves will result in oropharyngeal dysphagia. Impairment of oropharyngeal function is more apt to affect transport of liquids rather than solids, but this is not always the case. As a rule, patients usually can identify oropharyngeal symptoms much more readily than they can define symptoms implicating the esophagus itself.

Motor function within the body of the esophagus is controlled by a complex mechanism that involves both the central nervous system and the autonomic nervous system. The former regulates motor function within the upper portion of the esophagus (the proximal 3 to 4 cm that is invested by striated muscle). What happens in this proximal segment during the act of swallowing is a continuation of oropharyngeal events. Distally, the autonomic nervous system takes control and continues the wave propagation through a process of receptive relaxation and sequential contraction of the smooth muscle. The peristaltic wave travels smoothly along the body of the esophagus, passing through a relaxed lower esophageal sphincter. The latter then closes after the wave has completed its progress through the esophagus.

In functional disorders of the esophagus, there is disruption of this well-ordered propagation. There may be complete loss of peristaltic function, or there may be intermittent localized contractile activity that impedes the transport of solids or liquids through the esophagus and gives rise to distressing symptoms. In addition, disordered motor activity may cause relative zones of resistance to bolus flow within the esophagus, often increasing intraluminal pressure to abnormal amplitudes, thus delaying emptying of the esophagus.

> *"Oropharyngeal impairment is more apt to affect transport of liquids than solids—in most cases."*

In conditions such as achalasia, there is failure of sphincter relaxation following deglutition, which may reflect (but not exclusively so) postganglionic denervation and consequent lack of primary peristalsis within the body of the esophagus.[2] The sphincter maintains a normal or elevated resting tone that requires a build-up of pressure by a hydrostatic column of food or fluid within the esophagus before it opens to allow transfer of esophageal content into the stomach. Dysphagia may also occur with variants of achalasia (e.g., "vigorous" achalasia or diffuse esophageal spasm) (Fig. 4–2). Delay or obstruction to transit within the esophagus is responsible for impaired emptying and eventual esophageal decompensation and dilatation.

Peptic inflammatory disease can cause overt distal esophageal stricture formation or, in some cases, can result in more subtle forms of noncompliance. The latter can occur without formation of a demonstrable ring or cicatrix and may be very difficult to elucidate except by carefully conducted fluoroscopy after the swallowing of a solid bolus. Rings and webs can occur in the proximal or distal esophagus and often defy diagnosis by routine, standard diagnostic techniques.

It is worthwhile to briefly discuss the difference between dysphagia—that is, true difficulty with swallowing—and the "globus" feeling of impending dysphagia. The latter is a symptom that the interviewer may elicit from the patient who classically, but not always, appears anxious or hysterical. Globus may be described as the feeling of "a hand around the throat," or "a lump in the throat," or the perception that "a swallow just won't go down." Curiously, globus may often be transiently relieved by swallowing. A barium swallow shows normal transit of substances through the oropharynx into the stomach. Often, the patient who describes this symptom exhibits a hysterical personality. However, one should not casually dismiss the symptom of globus. Globus-like symptoms

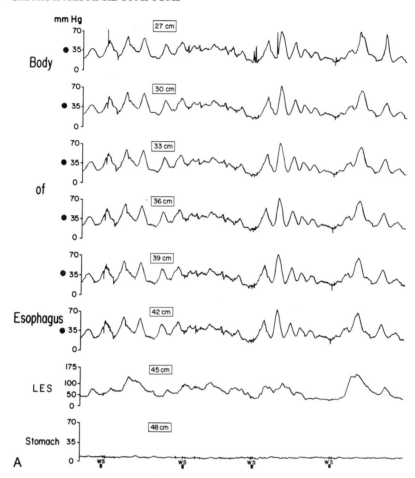

mm Hg

Body

of

Esophagus

LES

Stomach

A

FIGURE 4-2. A, *Vigorous achalasia.* Esophageal manometric tracing with recording tips in the body of the esophagus and the stomach. The lower esophageal sphincter (LES) pressure was recorded using a Dent sleeve sensor. Following water swallows (WS) there is a continuum of simultaneous common cavity motor activity throughout the esophageal body. Note that the LES pressure is elevated and there is little, if any, relaxation with swallows. B, *Diffuse esophageal spasm.* Esophageal manometric tracing showing disordered motor activity following initiation of a swallow. The second WS caused repetitive, high-amplitude contractions (spasm) that reached peak pressures of 600 mm Hg in the lower esophagus.

may sometimes herald an organic lesion and dysfunction of the upper eso-phageal sphincter or supraesophageal area is a possibility in this clinical condition.[3]

Features of oropharyngeal dysphagia include a change in vocal tone, a "garbled" voice, coughing during swallowing (particularly when drinking fluids), and choking while eating. Similar symptoms may occur during the night when the patient is unable to swallow oral secretions properly. There may be muscular weakness of the face or elsewhere in the body, dysarthria, and

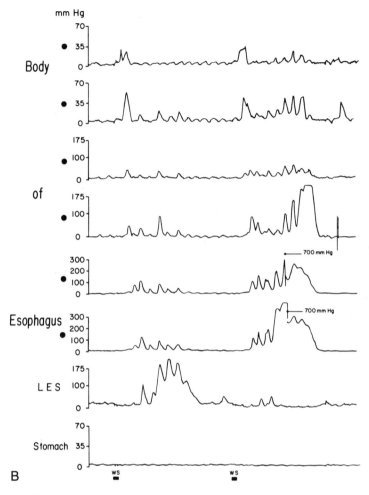

FIGURE 4.2 B   *Continued*

nasopharyngeal regurgitation. The last symptom is particularly devastating and often occurs when the patient attempts to drink fluids rapidly. There may be a so-called "labial spill" caused by weakness of the facial muscles, especially toward the end of the day.[4] Fluids may be tolerated best by sipping rather than gulping. On occasion, the patient may complain of being unable to suck or whistle. The patient may be frustrated by having to "chew, chew, chew" before attempts to swallow solids prove successful.

The patient with dysphagia referable to the body of the esophagus may complain that a food bolus, once swallowed, "slows down, sticks, or stops" (Table 4–1). Frequently, the patient will point to an area immediately beneath the lower sternum as the level of obstruction. It should be noted, however, that

TABLE 4-1.   The Three S's of Dysphagia

Do swallowed substances

- slow down?
- stick?
- stop?

an impacted food bolus within the esophagus may give symptoms referable to either the retrosternal area or the level of the suprasternal notch. The sensation of distress at the suprasternal notch, therefore, is not discriminating; it may imply the possibility of obstruction anywhere along the course of the esophagus.[5]

> "*Globus is typically seen in the overly anxious patient, but it should not be dismissed casually.*"

Patients with obstructive dysphagia can become quite sensitive to movement of material within the esophagus. They may describe "gurgling" and the sense of a pressure level that dissipates when the esophagus empties. Patients with profound motor disorders, such as achalasia, tend to drink water with each bolus of food. This serves to raise hydrostatic pressure sufficiently to effect esophageal emptying. The patient with achalasia also learns a series of maneuvers that can facilitate swallowing, such as hyperextending the neck so as to stretch the esophagus between its anatomic attachments and efface it as much as possible. In extreme cases of achalasia, patients may stand up, pound their chest, or raise their arms above their head. I have seen a few patients who admitted to actually jumping up and down at the dinner table to help to empty the esophagus.

The normal belch reflex may be impaired in achalasia. Patients frequently are unable to belch normally and volunteer that they now have only a "hollow, brief belch," not equivalent to the eructations of which they were capable in the past. This sort of feeble belch suggests eructation from the esophagus rather than from the stomach.[6] Symptoms of aspiration and choking are common in the patient with achalasia and indicate that the esophagus is no longer able to empty effectively or to prevent materials from spilling into the trachea.

The patient with diffuse esophageal spasm classically experiences obstructive dysphagia for food or fluid during the first few bites of the meal. At those times, the patient may excuse himself or herself from the table, regurgitate or vomit whatever he or she has tried to swallow, and then return to eat without further difficulty.[7] Cold substances, such as iced beverages, sometimes provoke this type of transient spasm, but occasionally a bolus of cold fluid may be sufficient to eliminate aggravating retrosternal distress. Chest pain and a stationary burning sensation are not uncommon in patients with diffuse esophageal motor disorders.[8] The burning has no orad component, as in classic pyrosis, and often is eliminated by ingestion of a bolus of water or a carbonated analgesic such as Alka-Seltzer.

Severe peptic esophagitis with noncompliance of the esophageal wall classically is associated with dysphagia for solids. Historically, the patient may indicate that he or she has difficulty in swallowing both liquids and solids. Close questioning, however, will determine that the patient first experiences solid bolus obstruction and that a subsequent attempt to ingest fluids is not only futile but also productive of regurgitation. Recurrent pneumonia, with or without symptoms of aspiration, may be the clinical presentation of the patient with achalasia. Surprisingly, a number of patients with achalasia present with a relatively indolent course. Periods of apparent obstructive dysphagia often are interspersed with intervals when swallowing is perceived as normal. Achalasia can be a longstanding condition marked by intermittently severe symptomatic expressions, similar to the clinical course of the celiac sprue syndrome.

Significance Within the Clinical Setting

Dysphagia and odynophagia mandate a response by the physician. These symptoms almost always indicate a significant, underlying health problem related to the patient's deglutitive mechanism. It is remarkable how often one sees patients with a clear-cut history of episodic dysphagia who have had repeatedly "normal" barium-meal examinations. Many times it will be found that the supposedly normal examination did not take into consideration the entire swallowing process from its inception in the oropharynx to the

"Questions pertaining to swallowing have to be properly phrased."

time of expulsion of contents through the esophagogastric junction. Within the clinical setting of dysphagia, an algorithm of questions pertaining to detailed features of the swallowing process needs to be developed to help the physician carefully assess some of the subtleties that may be absent or blurred because of the confluence of processes that occur when the swallowing mechanism is impaired.

Occasionally in clinical practice, when patients with overt peptic strictures narrowing the lumen of the esophagus to 2 mm or less are asked "Do you have problems swallowing?" the response is "No." If one rephrases the question as "Are you swallowing the same today as you did 2 years ago?" the same patient immediately protests "No, as a matter of fact, I'm not." Because of this experience, I now ask my questions about dysphagia in this sequence: "Do you experience trouble swallowing? Is your swallowing the same as it was 2 years ago?"

Odynophagia, on the other hand, is a complaint readily enunciated by the patient, probably because it usually is more acute in onset and often severe in intensity. This symptom not only alerts the patient and the physician, but it also demands prompt relief of the distress.

The differential diagnosis of oropharyngeal dysphagia ranges from cerebrovascular accidents, midbrain tumors, and cranial nerve disorders to neuromuscular impairments, such as myasthenia gravis and oropharyngeal dystrophy. Certain collagen-vascular diseases (e.g., polymyositis), iatrogenic radiation injury, and oropharyngeal tumors can cause dysphagia and painful swallowing. The latter symptom is a common feature of an oropharyngeal tumor before its presence is otherwise detected. There are a number of inflammatory processes that interfere with oropharyngeal deglutition. The question of hypertension or premature closure of the upper esophageal sphincter is only now being unraveled.[9]

Rings, strictures, pseudodiverticula, and other structural abnormalities may involve the body of the esophagus. In addition, loss of compliance may occur in localized areas of the esophagus (e.g., adjacent to the aortic arch) and sometimes may present with recurrent episodes of solid bolus obstruction. Segmental loss of esophageal compliance is often difficult to detect by conventional endoscopic and radiographic diagnostic techniques. One can only assume that subtle erosive peptic disease or perhaps ischemia may be the cause of muscular noncompliance in the upper half of the esophagus. This syndrome usually presents in younger persons. Multiple esophageal rings, some of which are extremely well developed, have been described as a cause of dysphagia.[10] Scleroderma, especially in association with hiatus hernia, can lead to severe peptic esophagitis, thereby aggravating the deleterious effect of the esophageal smooth muscle sclerosis.[11]

Primary esophageal motor disorders come in a variety of shades. Achalasia of the esophagus is the most classic form of primary motor disorder, although variations such as "vigorous achalasia" and diffuse esophageal spasm (perhaps a close relative) can cause severe problems with eating. The "nutcracker" esophagus has been much touted as a cause of intermittent dysphagia as well as other symptoms referable to the gullet.[12] This is a condition in which hypertensive esophageal contractions supposedly provoke pain, transient dysphagia, or both. The condition is probably similar to the hypertensive lower esophageal syndrome or the "tender esophagus."[13] The latter is associated with mild-to-moderate odynophagia with ingestion of a solid bolus and usually is seen in the very anxious patient. Scleroderma may present clinically as suspected achalasia because of its destructive effect upon the esophageal wall muscular tone and the lower esophageal sphincter. A variety of neuromuscular disorders, ranging from diabetic neuropathy to Parkinson's disease, may be associated with dysphagia. Interference with swallowing in such disorders, however, is a minor problem compared with the devastating effects on other organ systems.

Key Clinical Points

The symptoms of dysphagia need to be analyzed in detail (Table 4–2). Dysphagia usually is regionalized, but when it is perceived in the supraesophageal area rather than in the lower body of the esophagus, anatomic discrimination may be impossible. The patient, during questioning, should literally be led through the act of eating and deglutition in an attempt to point to the specific area of trouble. The physician needs to know whether the particular problem has occurred before, whether it is progressive, and whether it involves solids or liquids or both.

Isolated episodes of obstructive dysphagia are often easier to qualify, compared with repetitive and progressive episodes of dysphagia that occur with achalasia. The "steakhouse syndrome" was not given its name by accident (Fig. 4–3). The middle-aged gourmand who rushes in distress from a restaurant to the emergency room following impaction of a poorly chewed bolus of steak is a familiar figure.[14] Often he or she can be prompted to recall a previous occurrence of a similar problem. Appropriate treatment can be instituted expeditiously if an appropriate history is obtained.

The patient with achalasia exhibits a number of unique clinical features, mentioned earlier. The habit of imbibing fluid with each bit of solid food is a notorious trait of the achalasia patient, as is the sensation of gurgling or borborygmus-like noises in the chest. The patient with achalasia often can tell a physician when his or her esophagus is "empty," even when the ability to

TABLE 4–2. Dysphagia Profile

D	Difficulty swallowing?
Y	Yesterday's eating vs. 2 years ago?
S	Solids, liquids, or both?
P	Pattern of events?
H	Heartburn history?
A	Area of sensation?
G	Gradual or sudden onset?
I	Interventional measures?
A	Adverse weight loss?

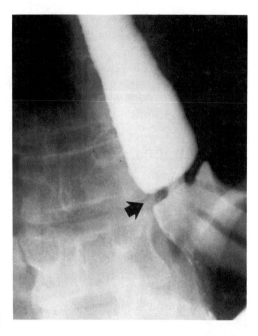

FIGURE 4-3. Barium-filled radiograph
demonstrating a well-developed Schatzki's ring
(*arrow*) above a hiatus hernia. The patient had been
admitted to the emergency room the week before for
an acute episode of "steakhouse syndrome" (see text)

perceive an individual food bolus has long ago disappeared. However, one of
the confusing features of far-advanced achalasia is that the patient no longer
appreciates the "fine tuning" associated with the swallowing process and
frequently is unaware of the extent to which swallowing has deteriorated
relative to normal, orderly deglutition.

> *"When questioning the patient, he or she
> should be led through the act of eating and
> deglutition, step by step."*

Upper esophageal rings are difficult to detect endoscopically and radiographically.[15] A history of difficulty in "getting down pills" is many times a
hallmark of an upper esophageal web or ring, as is a past history of occasional
dysphagia for solid foods.

A history of previous or concurrent heartburn is extremely important in
evaluating patients with dysphagia. As previously emphasized, true heartburn
is a perception of retrosternal burning with an orad-radiating component. It
can be expressed clinically in a number of diverse forms ranging from mild

retrosternal discomfort to angina-like chest pain extending to the neck, teeth, and interscapular back (see Chapter 3, "Heartburn").

Patients with primary esophageal motor disorders frequently describe a sense of "burning" that suggests gastroesophageal reflux, and this is an apparent paradox in the setting of achalasia. Such burning discomfort is believed to be secondary to stasis, esophageal dilatation, and purposeless contractile activity—not acid reflux.

The frequency, severity, and evolution of "classic" heartburn is sometimes a diagnostic clue to the underlying condition. Dysphagia caused by an esophageal stricture or supervening carcinoma in a columnar-lined (Barrett's) esophagus may be observed in a clinical setting wherein heartburn, once present, has gradually disappeared in more recent years.[16] Only when prompted may the patient recall troublesome heartburn in earlier decades of life. It has been suggested that this phenomenon is related to the transition from a squamous to a less sensitive columnar-lined Barrett's mucosa, or to an underlying malignant transformation.

A symptom significant of supraesophageal disorders is pharyngonasal regurgitation.[17] This is the backlash of liquid from a nonreceptive oropharynx out through the nose following ingestion of a fluid bolus. While this symptom strongly suggests supraesophageal or oropharyngeal impairment, intermittent esophageal spasm and upper esophageal sphincter relaxation can be associated with retropulsion of contents from the esophagus into the mouth. Even though this is a rare occurrence, there can be overlap of similar symptoms in disease processes as anatomically distinct as these examples.

The nervous patient is most difficult to assess when he or she presents with the symptoms of dysphagia. One may be able to obtain a history of transient slowing of a solid bolus during swallowing, which fulfills the criteria of dysphagia. Seldom do these patients have episodes of actual obstructive dysphagia, but they may have an annoying "bolus awareness" associated with a hypertensive esophageal contractile mechanism or a heightened afferent sensory apparatus (the "tender esophagus").

Odynophagia, as pointed out earlier, is a severe "hurting" during swallowing. With an acutely inflamed esophagus, not only does it hurt to swallow but pain on attempting to swallow may be so intense as to make swallowing impossible. Some of the most severe instances of odynophagia occur in patients who have "pill-induced" esophagitis complicated by edema and ulceration of the esophagus at its natural points of narrowing—that is, at the impingement by the aortic arch or at a site several centimeters above the esophagogastric junction.[18] Both are locations notorious for medication-related injuries. These patients may sometimes experience esophageal pain that lasts for months after apparent healing of the pill-induced esophagitis. Odynophagia is an occasional complaint of the patient whose esophagus has been recently dilated with filiform mercury-filled bougies. The shearing forces exerted by these instruments can deeply traumatize the intramural esophagus.[19] Patients who have had this type of dilation for noncompliant esophageal stricture or rings often require prolonged observation in the endoscopy holding area or overnight hospitalization because of severe odynophagia.

Finally, peptic esophagitis can cause odynophagia when ulceration is extensive enough to affect the deeper tissues of the esophagus. Some of the worst varieties of erosive and ulcerative esophagitis occur in patients with scleroderma or achalasia that has been complicated by gastroesophageal reflux disease. Potentially corrosive gastric contents entering the esophagus in these patients are not cleared and dissipated by the normal mechanisms, and the consequence is deep, longitudinal, erosive ulceration. Such lesions are often associated with intractable odynophagia and interscapular back pain.

Diagnostic Procedures

There are four important diagnostic steps in the evaluation of any patient with dysphagia or odynophagia:

1. A scrupulously taken history.
2. Perspicacious contrast fluoroscopy and radiography.
3. Careful endoscopy.
4. Manometric recording.

The history remains the foremost diagnostic tool. Information elicited from the patient helps point to the region of the pharynx or esophagus affected and sometimes suggests a specific cause toward which further diagnostic studies can be directed for confirmation.

> **"A** perceptive history is essential to the discriminating choice of further diagnostic tests."

The appropriate follow-up of a detailed history for a patient with a swallowing problem is real-time monitoring and recording of a barium swallow study performed by an experienced radiologist who is thoroughly knowledgeable about swallowing dynamics.[20] Too often, the inexperienced or disinterested radiologist begins to examine the course of a contrast medium in the esophagus only after the bolus is transported beyond the upper esophageal sphincter. Essential information may thus be lost. The advent of the "swallowgram" (including the triphasic study in which separate boluses of liquid, semisolid, and solid consistencies are sequentially observed) and new information derived from research on oropharyngeal swallowing mechanisms have helped to illuminate a heretofore obscure area of clinical medicine.

Observation of the formation of the bolus, its transmission through the oropharynx, the presence or absence of penetration into the airway, and the function of the upper esophageal sphincter yields information essential to anyone dealing with esophageal problems. A proper fluoroscopic and radiographic study includes attention to the presence or absence of effective peristalsis, structural distortion in the esophageal lumen, segments of stricture or noncompliance, and abnormality of esophageal caliber.

Most important and easily applicable is fluoroscopic observation supplemented by radiographic recordings of the passage of a barium-impregnated marshmallow through the esophagus after it has been swallowed. This method of study may be viewed as a sine qua non for assessing transport of a solid through the esophagus. Especially helpful is the observation of the level at which the barium-impregnated marshmallow may lodge or become impacted within the esophagus. We frequently make a diagnosis of localized esophageal noncompliance, ring formation, or mild stricture simply by performing this essential marshmallow-transit study. So often we have had patients referred with intermittent obstructive dysphagia for solids in whom a precise diagnosis could have been made earlier had this simple study been performed.

Esophagogastroscopy can divulge a great deal of information and provide objective evidence of active or chronic inflammation of the esophageal lining. Telltale marks of surface "pocketing," pseudodiverticula, and scars from chronic peptic esophagitis are best appreciated at endoscopy. Barrett's columnar-lined esophagus can be detected only by endoscopic examination and proven only by tissue biopsy. The esophagogastric junction of the patient with achalasia is best evaluated by endoscopy.[21] Symmetric effacement of a pliable sphincteric zone during insertion of the endoscope is valuable information. Obtaining a view of the gastroesophageal junction from below, by retroflexion of the endoscope, is crucial in excluding an infiltrative process or other structural abnormality that might present as "pseudo-achalasia." However, one should be mindful that endoscopy is not a sensitive method for detecting subtle motor impairment of the pharynx or esophagus.

Esophageal manometry is a uniquely useful diagnostic technique for establishing a primary esophageal motor disorder. With the introduction of the Dent sleeve sensor, sphincter pressure and relaxation can now be monitored despite axial movement caused by respiration or swallowing.[22] The standard water-perfused esophageal manometry catheter assembly is an excellent tool for measuring the propagation and magnitude of peristalsis throughout the body of the esophagus; however, it does not record pressure events in the oropharynx with fidelity. A sleeve sensor placed in the upper esophageal sphincter, combined with several miniaturized solid-state pressure transducers, can give an excellent profile of pressure events and their sequence within the oropharynx.[23]

Concurrent esophageal manometry and videofluoroscopy allow an image-to-image comparison of esophageal events and flow dynamics and provide a unique and accurate assessment of severe motor disorders. Combined sequencing by this means in patients with gross motor defects of the esophagus associated with epiphrenic diverticula, diffuse esophageal spasm, and noncompliant zones of the esophagus yields invaluable information otherwise impossible to obtain. In addition, we are only beginning to learn about factors such as relative resistance to flow within the esophagus, which increases intraluminal pressure and affects transmission of peristalsis in the proximal esophagus.[24] I believe that this phenomenon can be clinically perceived and transcribed into symptoms of dysphagia and, occasionally, odynophagia.

To Sum Up

The symptoms of dysphagia and odynophagia should sound a significant alarm to the clinician. These symptoms imply a serious problem with the transport mechanism that may involve one or many complex structural and functional mechanisms within the swallowing apparatus. The occurrence of these symptoms requires an explanation on every occasion by the physician; invariably an underlying problem is initiating these target-specific symptoms. The purported absence of positive findings in "standard" diagnostic studies should not deter the clinician from continuing to pursue an answer to the problem. The solution may require more sophisticated diagnostic techniques or perhaps consultation with someone who is especially experienced and concerned in this area of gastroenterology. First and foremost, the search for an explanation of dysphagia and odynophagia requires a very specific, detailed, and exhaustive history of all aspects of the patient's swallowing difficulties. Not only will this improve the diagnostic yield, but it also will be found cost-effective.

References

1. Kahrilas PJ. The anatomy and physiology of dysphagia. In: Gelfand DW, Richter JE, eds. Dysphagia: Diagnosis and treatment, New York: Igaku-Shoin 1989:110–128.
2. Vantrappen G, Janssens J, Helemens J, et al. Achalasia, diffuse esophageal spasm and related motility disorders. Gastroenterology 1979; 76:450–457.
3. Cook IJ, Shaker R, Dodds WJ, et al. Role of mechanical and chemical stimulation of the esophagus in globus sensation. Gastroenterology 1989 (abstract); 96(5):A99.
4. Curtis DJ, Cruess DF, Dachman DH. Normal erect swallowing: Normal function and incidence of variations. Invest Radiol 1985; 20:717–726.
5. Castell DO. Dysphagia. Gastroenterology 1979; 76:1015–1024.
6. Massey BT, Hogan WJ, Dodds WJ, Dantas RO. Impairment of the esophageal belch reflex in achalasia patients: Abnormality of the upper esophageal sphincter response. Gastroenterology 1989 (abstract); 96:5.
7. Richter JE, Castell DO. Diffuse esophageal spasm: A reappraisal. Ann Intern Med 1984; 100:242–245.

8. Smart HL, Foster PN, Evans DF, et al. Twenty-four hour oesophageal acidity in achalasia before and after pneumatic dilatation. Gut 1987; 28:883–887.
9. Cook IJ, Dodds WJ, Dantas R, et al. Opening mechanisms of the human upper esophageal sphincter. Am J Physiol 1989; 257:6748–6759.
10. Shifle HDW, Gelliam JH, Wu WC, et al. Multiple esophageal webs. Gastroenterology 1979; 77:556–559.
11. Venu R, Hogan WJ, Geenen JE, et al. Complications of gastroesophageal reflux in scleroderma: High risk factors associated with esophageal stricture. Gastrointest Endosc 1980 (abstract); 26(2):79.
12. Katz PO, Dalton CB, Richter JE, et al. Esophageal testing in patients with noncardiac chest pain and/or dysphagia. Ann Intern Med 1987; 106:593–597.
13. Edwards DA. Discriminatory value of symptoms in the differential diagnosis of dysphagia. Clin Gastroenterol 1976; 5:49–57.
14. Glancy JJ, Spiro HM. Lower esophageal ring. N Engl J Med 1970; 292:1292–1305.
15. Ekbery O, Malmquest J, Lindren S. Pharyngo-oesophageal webs in dysphageal patients—a radiological and clinical investigation in 1134 patients. Fortschr Rontgenstr 1986; 145:75–80.
16. Spechler SJ, Goyal RK. Barrett's esophagus. N Engl J Med 1986; 315:362–371.
17. Castell DO. Dysphagia: A general approach to the patient. In: Gelfand DW, Richter JE, eds. Dysphagia: Diagnosis and treatment. New York: Igaku-Shoin, 1989:3–9.
18. Kikendell JW, Friedman AC, Oyawole MA, et al. Pill-induced esophageal injury. Dig Dis Sci 1983; 28:174–182.
19. Tulman AB, Boyce HW. Complications of esophageal dilatation and guidelines for their prevention. Gastrointest Endosc 1981; 27:229–234.
20. Curtis PJ, Cruess DF, Wellgress FR. Abnormal solid bolus swallowing in erect position. Dysphagia 1987; 2:46–49.
21. Kahrilas PJ, Kishk SM, Helm JF, et al. Comparison of pseudoachalasia and achalasia. Am J Med 1987; 82:439–440.
22. Dent J. A new technique for continuous sphincter pressure measurements. Gastroenterology 1976; 71:9–15.
23. Shaker R, Cook IJ, Dodds WJ, Hogan WJ. Pressure-flow dynamics of the oral phase of swallowing. Dysphagia 1988; 3:79–84.
24. Massey BT, Dodds WJ, Hogan WJ, et al. Abnormal esophageal motility: Comparison of radiographic and manometric findings. Gastroenterology 1988 (abstract); 95(3):879.

NAUSEA AND VOMITING

William S. Haubrich, M.D.

5

Nausea is a symptom; vomiting, when witnessed, is a sign. Both can be helpful by their presence or absence, in assessing the state of a patient with a digestive problem. Both can be guides to a discriminating choice of tests that, in most cases, will lead to a diagnosis and, hence, to appropriate management.

Much is known, yet much remains to be discovered, of the nature of nausea and vomiting. In brief, the mechanism of nausea and vomiting involves a central vomiting center in the dorsal part of the lateral reticular formation of the medulla oblongata. This well-defined center lies in close association with the respiratory center and an array of nuclei that relate to various visceral functions, such as salivation and defecation. It is also near centers having to do with vestibular and vasomotor functions. While distinct, these centers are liable to spill-over of stimuli from one to another and, as will be discussed, symptoms and signs relating to several of the centers may be concomitant and mixed. There is not, so far as known, a distinct nausea center. Probably the symptom of nausea results from early and subliminal stimulation of the vomiting center.

Afferent impulses arising from a variety of sources throughout the organism can converge on the vomiting center where, depending on their intensity, they can be translated into effector impulses that activate or inhibit visceral and peripheral structures. For example, the presence in the stomach of a substance disagreeable to the gastric mucosa can stimulate impulses mediated mainly by vagal afferent fibers that are directed to the vomiting center. Reception of these impulses, as perceived and integrated by the vomiting center, may then induce efferent impulses mediated along autonomic pathways to gastroenteric smooth muscle and to associated effector structures that result in retrograde emptying of the proximal alimentary tract. This, of course, is a reflex arc that can be completed, depending on the need, in a matter of seconds. Often, however, the interval between initiation of afferent impulses and their translation to effector organs is much more protracted.

"There is a central vomiting center, but no known equivalent nausea center."

How to Inquire of the Nature of Nausea and Vomiting

Nausea is often difficult for the patient to describe and sometimes difficult for the clinician to assay. The patient may not even use the word. Often he or she says simply, "I feel sick." Linguistically, "sick" was at one time equivalent to "nauseated," and this use persists when the patient says, "I think I'm going to be sick." The patient really is trying to say, "I feel waves of nausea, and I think I'm going to throw up." This is an anticipation of vomiting and should prompt the physician or nurse to reach for a handy emesis basin.

When patients try to describe nausea, they often say, "It's the feeling I have before I vomit." But nausea is by no means always a prelude to vomiting. It can be—and often is—a freestanding symptom, especially when it is a recurrent or chronic complaint. Nausea has been aptly described as a *forme fruste* of vomiting.

An occasional patient will describe nausea as the disagreeable feeling they have had when seasick, if seasickness has been a past experience. Indeed, the very word "nausea" has a nautical connection. Both "nausea" and "nautical" share a common origin in the Greek word *naus,* meaning "a ship." The ancient Greeks gave the term *nausia* to the ill feeling they associated with the rolling and pitching of their seagoing ships.

Another word that patients sometimes use, especially for milder forms of nausea that may not culminate in vomiting, is "queasy." This usually refers to a generally unsettled feeling; or some patients may say they have an "all gone feeling." If asked to indicate where they feel nausea or queasiness, patients usually place a hand on the epigastrium or sometimes on the throat.

As with all symptoms, it is of first importance to establish the duration of nausea. The general rule applies: the likelihood of finding a discoverable cause for the symptom is inversely related to its duration. The longer the duration, the less likely will be a confirmed cause; conversely, the shorter the duration, the more assiduous should be the search for a provocative lesion.

Next in importance is to determine whether nausea has been accompanied by actual vomiting. In response to this question, some patients will be evasive: "Well, I have this bad taste in my mouth." This, of course, is not vomiting. Longstanding nausea combined with a "bad taste" in the mouth is almost a sure clue to a chronically depressed state. Any attempt to find a lesion in the mouth or in the alimentary canal will likely prove futile. The patient may say, "Well, I burp a lot." This is hardly helpful. Most, if not all, patients with nausea of more than mild degree are air-swallowers (see Chapter 12, "Gaseousness"). They swallow air because of hypersalivation that often accompanies nausea and because nausea by itself many times is a subliminal stimulus to "dry swallows."

The patient may mention "acid brash" (i.e., a sense of sour fluid welling up in the back of the throat). This, of course, is a symptom of gastroesophageal reflux and often, but not necessarily, attends hiatus hernia (see Chapter 3, "Heartburn"). Nausea, however, is not a common symptom of hiatus hernia, and only rarely does the patient with uncomplicated peptic ulcer disease complain of nausea. Nausea as a new symptom voiced by a peptic ulcer patient points to a complication, usually gastric stasis due to obstruction or, in some cases, bleeding.

Nausea in the absence of vomiting almost always is of central rather than peripheral origin. That is to say, it is initiated centrally in the brain rather than peripherally in the alimentary tract. This form of nausea, whether of long or short duration, is more likely to be a response to a metabolic disorder (e.g., azotemia) or a reflection of disturbance in higher cortical centers (e.g., witnessing a repugnant scene). Testimony to the latter is given in common expressions such as "That sort of behavior makes me sick," or "I feel sick just thinking about it." "Sick," as expressed here and as previously noted, is equivalent or akin to nausea.

> "*Nausea in the absence of vomiting almost always is of central rather than peripheral origin.*"

Vomiting has to be seen to be appreciated. Many patients' description of vomiting tends to be exaggerated in terms of violence, volume, and frequency. It is remarkable how often patients confuse rumination, regurgitation, acid brash, or even mere water brash with actual vomiting. Rumination is the process of chewing cud (i.e., bringing back into the mouth whatever has been previously swallowed), an act normal to cows, sheep, goats, deer, and giraffes, but seen only rarely, as an aberrant symptom, in humans (see Chapter 14 "Eating Disorders"). Regurgitation is similar but usually involuntary; what fills the mouth by retrograde propulsion is often the contents of the esophagus, but it can include stomach contents as well. Typically, regurgitation is not associated with nausea and is less rigorous than vomiting. Acid brash, which, as previously mentioned, is a welling up in the throat or mouth of sour gastric juice, signifies an incompetent lower esophageal sphincter mechanism, and it may or may not be attended by nausea. Water brash is an outpouring in the mouth of tasteless serous or mucoid fluid, mostly saliva. Often the patient will spit out this fluid, but this is not vomiting. However, water brash is commonly associated with nausea, often as a prelude to actual vomiting.

A key question is whether vomiting was preceded by nausea. In most cases the answer will be yes. However, vomiting in the absence of nausea, especially vomiting that occurs abruptly or "out of the blue" and that is exceptionally violent or "explosive," can be an ominous sign. In such instances the vomiting is often indicative of a lesion in the brain, such as a tumor, that may cause elevated intracranial pressure. Vomiting of similar type may also be encountered in infants with hypertrophic pyloric stenosis.

Vomiting preceded by "gut rumbling" or colicky abdominal pain suggests, of course, obstruction of the alimentary tract, particularly in the intestine. Because the small intestine does not tolerate distention, the interval between obstruction of the small intestine and vomiting is much less than that in cases of distal colon obstruction. In the former case, the duration of antecedent colicky pain may be only minutes or hours; in the latter case, the interval may be as long as several days.

Vomiting attended by symptoms of hypovolemia, such as lassitude, sunken eyes, pallor, and poor skin turgor, bespeaks depletion of large volumes of fluid and electrolytes.

Vomiting preceded or followed by diarrhea, especially when acute, suggests widespread gastroenteric irritation, commonly due to infection, typically that by a virus.

In the absence of witnessed vomiting, the clinician is obliged to do the best he or she can to estimate the amount and character of the emesis from the patient's account. Whenever possible, it is always helpful to examine the emesis. The emesis basin should always be intercepted for inspection by the physician before its contents are discarded by the nurse. Of first importance is the volume. Is the bottom of the emesis basin merely moistened by a few drops of spittle, or is the basin overflowing? Are there recognizable food particles, or does the fluid consist of what appears to be gastric juice? Is the emesis stained by bile or blood? If there is blood, is it bright red, maroon, brown, or black? The odor of emesis fluid should be noted. When unusually fetid, the emesis may be of long-retained gastric contents. A feculent appearance or odor may suggest the possibility of a gastrocolic fistula.

Vomiting is generally of two types: irritative or retentive. The former is much more frequent than the latter. Irritative vomiting may be provoked by ingestion of food or fluid, or it may occur at any time between meals or during the night. The vomitus consists of whatever was in the stomach at the time: ingested food or fluid, or simply gastric juice and ropy mucus. If irritative vomiting is provoked immediately after eating, undigested food consumed shortly before vomiting is readily recognized in the vomitus. Ask the patient how the vomitus tasted. Food or fluid regurgitated from an obstructed esophagus has little or no taste; gastric juice tastes sour, except in cases of markedly diminished or absent gastric acid secretion. Irritative vomiting, when severe, often leads to rigorous retching. The empty stomach convulses, but there is little or nothing to come up. This may be described by the patient as "dry heaves."

---

*"**A** key question is whether vomiting was preceded by nausea."*

Retentive vomiting, as the emesis of long-accumulated gastric contents, such as occurs in cases of pyloric obstruction, is recognized by vomitus of large volume and by the presence of long-retained, partially digested food particles. This is illustrated by the following dialogue:

Physician: What did you vomit?
Patient: The funny thing is that I vomited watermelon seeds.
Physician: What's so funny about that?
Patient: I haven't eaten watermelon since 3 days ago.

One is mindful that an emesis of long-retained gastric contents does not always mean obstruction at the pylorus or duodenum. It simply means impaired gastric emptying, and this is seen also in cases of gastric paresis in the absence of gastric outlet obstruction. An example is the sluggish stomach that sometimes complicates longstanding diabetes. A caveat: one should be extremely cautious in proposing a diagnosis of gastroparesis diabeticorum in the absence of other signs of diabetic neuropathy, such as orthostatic hypotension. Also, it is helpful to remember that some elderly patients, more often women, seem to acquire, among the ravages of age, large, baggy, hypotonic stomachs that sometimes empty the wrong way.

The presence of bile in vomitus is often not as significant as it may seem. One might think that vomiting bile-stained fluid points to an obstructing lesion in the duodenum distal to the entry of the common bile duct. Not so. Normally, bile regurgitates from the duodenum into the stomach sufficient to stain vomitus from almost any cause. An absence of bile in retentive vomitus might suggest obstruction at or proximal to the pylorus; an unusually heavy load of bile in postprandial vomiting might suggest the afferent loop syndrome in a patient who has had a gastrojejunostomy. But, again, one should expect some bile staining in any sort of emesis.

The presence of visible blood in vomitus is another matter (see Chapter 6, "Gastrointestinal Bleeding"). This is often, but not always, significant. A few streaks of fresh red blood tainting mucoid vomitus probably is the result of retching, coming from abrasion of small mucosal vessels in the esophagus or pharynx. This need not be a cause for alarm. Larger amounts of fresh blood, especially that emitted after a paroxysm of rigorous retching, may signify a Mallory-Weiss tear in the mucosa at the esophagogastric junction. In most cases, this sort of bleeding, even though disturbing at first sight, subsides spontaneously. Nevertheless, careful observation is in order. Relatively fresh blood, in volume, vomited by a patient with evidence of liver disease, suggests a source in ruptured esophageal varices.

Blood exposed to gastric acid quickly darkens. Hence, altered blood in vomitus (i.e., blood darkened by exposure to gastric acid) points to a bleeding source below the esophagogastric junction, usually from erosions or ulcerations in the gastroduodenal mucosa. Blood, of course, must be exposed to acid to turn dark. Large volumes of blood from a profusely bleeding source, even from an acid-secreting stomach, will appear largely red because the blood is quickly vomited and hence inadequately exposed to gastric acid (see Chapter 6).

What has been said in the preceding paragraphs about vomited blood also applies to the inspection of blood in gastric contents aspirated through a nasogastric tube, whether the tube has been only just introduced or has been indwelling. In any case, it is visible blood that counts. It is fatuous to test either vomitus or an aspirate from a nasogastric tube for occult blood. It is almost impossible to aspirate through a tube or to vomit with force and not have the fluid contain a modicum of blood sufficient to test positively with benzidine or guaiac. If blood cannot be seen with the eye in such material, ignore it.

A proclivity to both nausea and vomiting varies strikingly from one person to another, for reasons that are not altogether clear. Some persons declare they frequently "feel sick" with what seems only slight provocation. Others claim never to have experienced nausea, even in what would be thought to be the most conducive circumstances. Therefore, the perspicacious physician is obliged to judge the significance of complaints of nausea and vomiting, or their absence, in this light. This is not always an easy task.

Moreover, tendencies to nausea and to vomiting do not necessarily go hand-in-hand. There are those who claim to have often felt deathly "sick at the stomach" yet say they have been unable to vomit, as hard as they may have tried. Presumably, such impaired persons are unable to coordinate the neuromuscular mechanism necessary for the act of vomiting. Similar impediment to vomiting can be seen in persons with a "cascade stomach," marked by exceptionally acute angulation at the esophagogastric junction, and also in patients who have had a previous surgical fundoplication. Other persons seemingly can empty their stomachs at will. They can and do vomit readily at the first inclination toward even mild nausea.

Nausea not only is typically a prelude to spontaneous vomiting but also, for some persons, a prompting to induce vomiting as a means of obtaining relief from their disagreeable symptom. Such a practice is sometimes observed in patients with peptic ulcer disease, who have found that a sizable reduction in gastric acid accomplished by induced vomiting temporarily relieves their distress. Oddly, it is not always easy to discern induced or spontaneous vomiting. Occasionally, a patient admits to inserting a finger in the throat to cause vomiting, but not always is this remembered or acknowledged. It may be of no matter; it cannot be said that spontaneous vomiting is necessarily more serious than induced vomiting.

Conditions Often Associated with Nausea and Vomiting

In considering other symptoms and signs frequently associated with nausea and vomiting, one has to bear in mind a reciprocal relationship; that is, nausea and vomiting in relation to other symptoms can be either cause or effect. A distinction is not always clear and, in some cases, both circumstances may pertain.

Vasomotor Responses.   Sweating, pallor, and hypotension often are observed in patients suffering intense nausea and vomiting, probably because of the proximity in the medulla of the vomiting center and nuclei that control various vasomotor responses. In general, such vasomotor responses reflect the acuity, but not necessarily the gravity, of the nausea and vomiting.

Pain.   Severe pain of any sort seems to provoke nausea and vomiting in some persons. Visceral pain—that is, pain transmitted along autonomic afferent pathways—is more likely to be attended by nausea and vomiting than

"Be aware that nausea or vomiting in a pain-wracked patient may be a side effect of medication taken to allay pain."

pain transmitted from the periphery along cerebrospinal pathways. Visceral pain tends to be a "sick pain," cutaneous or musculoskeletal pain less so. For example, pain arising in pancreatitis is much more likely to be attended by nausea and vomiting than pain of similar intensity arising from a broken leg. Acutely painful pancreatitis or calculous biliary tract disease are two conditions notoriously associated with repeated, sometimes almost incessant, vomiting.

Be aware, however, that nausea or vomiting in a pain-wracked patient may be side effects of medication taken to allay pain.

Labyrinthine Disturbances. Labyrinthine disturbances notoriously are marked by nausea and vomiting. This is commonly seen in cases of *mal de mer* (seasickness). The associated symptom is true vertigo, not merely lightheadedness. Another well-known example is Ménière's syndrome. Conversely, nausea and vomiting in some persons commonly is associated with what the patient describes as "dizziness," but what is really giddiness or lightheadedness. Dizziness not characterized as true vertigo, when it accompanies nausea and vomiting, is not likely to be caused by a labyrinthine disorder.

Pregnancy. Among women in their childbearing years, "morning sickness" of pregnancy may account for their experience with nausea and vomiting. Documentation of the menstrual history is essential in the evaluation of any woman complaining of nausea or vomiting. (This is important, if for no other reason, to avoid exposing a possibly pregnant woman to diagnostic radiography.) It is surprising how many young women may be unaware of an early pregnancy, the first sign of which can be "morning sickness." This benign, although disagreeable, condition typically is confined to the first trimester of pregnancy. More serious is hyperemesis gravidarum, which can plague a woman throughout her pregnancy. Still more grave, and commonly attended by prostrating nausea and vomiting, is eclampsia occurring in the last trimester of pregnancy.

Drugs and Chemicals. Numerous drugs and chemicals are well known to induce nausea and vomiting. Probably the most frequent offender is alcohol, especially in young persons whose tolerance is low. Also, nausea and vomiting frequently are part of the daily experience of the chronic alcoholic. As mentioned previously, analgesic drugs, especially those of the opiate genre, regularly induce nausea and vomiting in susceptible persons. Often the patient is aware of this diathesis from previous experience. The thoughtful physician inquires of such idiosyncrasies before prescribing anodynes.

Among other offending drugs (the list is almost endless) are the cardiotonic agents, such as digitalis and quinidine (in any of their forms). Nausea and vomiting are almost invariable concomitants of many of the agents used in cancer chemotherapy. Finally, there are some compulsive patients who regularly consult their own copy of the Physicians' Desk Reference whenever they are given a prescription. Almost invariably they will find nausea and vomiting listed among the possible side effects of the medication they are supposed to take; this, then, can become a self-fulfilling prophecy.

Metabolic Disorders. Metabolic disorders often are attended by nausea and vomiting, although the exact mechanisms are not always clear. A prime example is azotemia resulting from advanced renal impairment. Another example is jaundice, especially that due to intrahepatic cholestasis. Hyperparathyroidism and hyperthyroidism are endocrine disorders in which nausea and vomiting are frequent features; adrenal insufficiency is another. In most cases, the underlying metabolic disturbance will be otherwise evident; in other cases, however, it may be hidden until a blood chemistry panel is obtained.

Respiratory Symptoms. Respiratory symptoms can be associated with nausea and vomiting. Chief among these is cough, especially when a barking cough occurs in violent paroxysms. The patient may say, "I coughed so hard, I threw up." The probable explanation is that the medullary vomiting center reverberates from impulses emanating from the nearby cough center. Occasionally, the retching predominates, and the antecedent cough is overlooked. Chronic sinusitis with postnasal "drip" and the wheezing of asthmatic bronchitis are often attended by nausea, if not vomiting. Here, again, inquiry about medication is important, inasmuch as many people find nausea a disagreeable side effect of ephedrine and other adrenergic drugs taken to relieve respiratory disorders.

Heart Disease. Heart disease, even in the patient not taking cardiotonic drugs, can be evident in nausea and vomiting. These are not symptoms usually associated with uncomplicated coronary artery insufficiency (although patients with angina pectoris tend to become air-swallowers), but vomiting as an accompaniment of severe retrosternal pain may signify a transmural myocardial infarct. The patient with acute right ventricular failure, as in mitral stenosis, may present with abrupt right upper quadrant pain (from sudden passive hyperemia in the liver), nausea, and vomiting that appear to mimic acute cholecystitis.

Brain Lesions. Mention has been made of the ominous abrupt nausea and explosive vomiting that can occur in patients with intracranial lesions. In this setting, a prompt and meticulous search for associated neurologic signs is mandatory.

Emotional Disturbance. Emotional disturbances, both acute and chronic, are well known to be expressed as nausea and vomiting. Panic attacks are often reflected in stomach upheaval. Anorexia, smoldering nausea, and even weight loss are commonly prominent among the symptoms of protracted depression.

Brief Guide to the Need for Further Tests

It is not usual for nausea and vomiting to occur in an otherwise total symptomatic vacuum. Preceding, concomitant, or subsequent associated symptoms and signs can be elicited in most patients, even those presenting with nausea or vomiting as a chief complaint. The key to further procedures is found in these

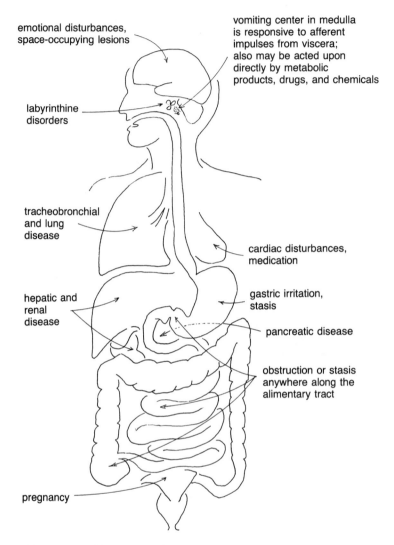

emotional disturbances,
space-occupying lesions

vomiting center in medulla
is responsive to afferent
impulses from viscera;
also may be acted upon
directly by metabolic
products, drugs, and chemicals

labyrinthine
disorders

tracheobronchial
and lung
disease

cardiac disturbances,
medication

hepatic and
renal
disease

gastric irritation,
stasis

pancreatic disease

obstruction or stasis
anywhere along the
alimentary tract

pregnancy

FIGURE 5-1. Some of the many sources of nausea and vomiting.

accompanying symptoms and signs. This is especially true when nausea and vomiting have been of recent onset (fig. 5-1).

The problem of the patient presenting with nausea or vomiting as a sole complaint requires a different tack. In most such cases, the complaint will have been protracted, and the patient, while distressed, will not likely be depleted. In such instances, there should be no precipitous rush to embark on a series of intensive or rigorous investigations. Moreover, when nausea and vomiting occur as the sole indication of acute gastroenteric irritation, the problem usually is self-limited, and the symptoms will abate before extensive tests can be undertaken.

Following a thorough physical examination (which usually will be unrevealing but may yield a clue to the need for a more specific search), it is appropriate to proceed with simple measures, such as urinalysis, hemogram, and blood chemistry panel. These may betray an occult anemia or metabolic derangement.

A scout film of the abdomen, while easily obtained, is seldom revealing except when there are associated symptoms suggesting obstruction. The same is true for barium-meal radiographic examination.

Endoscopy of the upper gastrointestinal tract is not likely to be helpful except in cases when nausea and vomiting are attended by signs of significant bleeding; then endoscopy is mandatory. One does well to bear in mind that endoscopy performed when the patient has been rigorously vomiting can be misleading. In such instances, the finding of a few mucosal erosions may only magnify an otherwise minor problem and lead to performance of still another, repeated examination to see if the trivial lesions have disappeared. Endoscopy is not always definitive in patients suspected of obstruction as a cause of vomiting; selection of contrast fluoroscopy and radiography is the better choice.

Ultrasonography, computed tomography (CT), and magnetic resonance imaging play no role in the case of the patient complaining of only nausea or vomiting, except in the special circumstance when an intracranial lesion is suspected. Then the choice is CT of the head, not of the abdomen.

Illustrative Case

A 32-year-old woman anxiously called in to arrange an urgent appointment because of increasing nausea over the preceding 2 days. Within hours of the onset of nausea, she had vomited several times, but because she had no appetite and had not eaten, the emesis was small and nondescript. She had no idea of what might have provoked her nausea; her genitourinary function was undisturbed.

When initially seen, the patient mentioned almost incidentally that she had also had pain but could not recall whether the nausea or the pain had come first. What was significant was that the pain, at first only a vague epigastric distress, had become sharply localized below the right costal margin. What was even more striking, on physical examination that was otherwise unremarkable, was that point tenderness with muscle guarding was elicited in the right upper quadrant of the abdomen just beneath the costal margin.

Urinalysis was clear. The hemogram was normal, except for a white blood cell count of 14,000, predominantly neutrophils. A scout film of the abdomen was unrevealing. After the point tenderness and muscle guarding in the right upper quadrant were confirmed by several observers, the patient was taken to surgery with a preoperative diagnosis of acute appendicitis, thought to be adjacent to a high-lying cecum.

This diagnosis, as revealed at operation, was not quite accurate. The patient was found to have an acutely inflamed, solitary diverticulum in the distal limb of the hepatic flexure of the colon. The appendix was uninvolved. The offending diverticulum was locally resected, and the patient's recovery was uneventful.

As the late Chester Jones was often quoted, "If you can't make a diagnosis, make a decision." Our initial diagnosis, based on the patient's symptoms and signs, had been a bit off the mark, but our decision for a needed operation was correct.

Comment.   This is hardly a typical case of a patient presenting with nausea and vomiting; but then there can hardly be a typical case, inasmuch as nausea and vomiting are masks behind which lurk a host of diverse disturbances.

In this case, what brought the problem into focus was the associated pain, which the patient nearly glossed over in recounting her symptoms. The importance of the pain was underscored by the finding of point tenderness and muscle guarding in the right upper abdominal quadrant. Bolstering the decision to intervene surgically was the elevated white blood cell count.

The finding of an isolated colonic diverticulitis at an unusual site was a surprise but by no means a disappointment, even though it refuted our presumptive diagnosis. The patient's problem was properly managed, and that was what mattered.

To Sum Up

The significance of nausea and vomiting is best assessed by meticulous history taking and physical examination. The perceptive physician quickly learns to judge the implications of the setting in which nausea and vomiting occur and the manner in which the patient describes his or her symptoms. Unless the acuity or severity of associated symptoms is compelling, symptomatic and supportive measures allow time for a thoughtful consideration of the need for further investigation.

Suggested Reading

Barksy AJ, Goodson JD, Lane RS. The amplification of somatic symptoms. Psychosom Med 1988; 50:510–519.

Borison HL, Wang SC. Physiology and pharmacology of vomiting. Pharmacol Rev 1953; 5:193–230.

Clearfield HB, Roth JLA. Anorexia, nausea, and vomiting. In: Berk JE, Haubrich WS, Kalser MH, Roth JLA, Schaffner F, eds. Bockus Gastroenterology. 4th ed. Philadelphia: WB Saunders, 1985:48–58.

Cleghorn RA, Brown WT. Psychogenesis of emesis. Can Psychiatric Assoc J 1964; 9:299–310.

Ingram DA, Fulton RA, Portal RW, Aber CP. Vomiting as a diagnostic aid in acute ischemic cardiac pain. Br Med J 1980; 281:636–637.

Lumsden K, Holden WS. The act of vomiting in man. Gut 1969; 10:173–179.

Schreirer L, Cutler RM, Saigal V. Vomiting as a dominant symptom of asthma. Ann Allergy 1987; 58:118–120.

Swanson DW, Swenson WM, Huizenga KA, Melson SJ. Persistent nausea without organic cause. Mayo Clin Proc 1976; 51:257–262.

GASTROINTESTINAL BLEEDING

Abraham Bogoch, M.D., B.Sc. (Med.), D.Sc.

6

The ability to determine precisely the cause of bleeding from the gastrointestinal tract is often difficult despite numerous technical advances in recent years. Nevertheless, information gained from a carefully taken history and the findings on physical examination will often suggest the locale as well as the likely cause for bleeding.

Examination of the vomitus and stool is essential to the basic clinical assessment of gastrointestinal bleeding. When the patient vomits blood, the source of bleeding is the esophagus, stomach, or duodenum in the large majority of cases. When truly tarry stools are passed, the site of bleeding is usually the same. Depending on the origin of bleeding, its volume, the intestinal transit time, and the bulk of residual feces in the intestine, stools may be described variously as bright red, magenta, dark cherry red, maroon, dark brownish red, black, or tarry. Relating color changes of the stool to the site of bleeding, although it is generally useful and reliable, may be misleading. For example, passage of bright red blood from the rectum can, in instances of exceptionally rapid transit, be the consequence of massive bleeding from a duodenal ulcer. Thus, the volume of bleeding and the intestinal transit time are sometimes as important as the site of bleeding in determining the color of a blood-laden stool passed from the rectum.

It seems obvious, yet merits a reminder, that if the patient's history is to be reliable, the patient must have actually observed his or her stools. Surprisingly, the following dialogue often ensues:

Physician: Have your stools been red or black?
Patient: No.
Physician: Have you looked at your stools?
Patient: Oh, no. I can never bear to look in the toilet bowl.

"Examination of vomitus and stool is essential in the clinical assessment of gastrointestinal bleeding."

Further, particularly when questioning men, one does well to ask if the patient is color-blind. A color-blind person cannot be expected to accurately discern the color of his or her stools.

Features of the history antecedent to bleeding will often help fix the site of bleeding to the upper or lower alimentary tract and may also provide a clue to its cause. Distinctly useful in assessing the severity of bleeding are certain findings on physical examination, which are summarized in Table 6–1.

In the sections that follow, bleeding from the digestive tract is classified for clarity of consideration into *hematemesis, melena,* and *hematochezia.*

Hematemesis

Hematemesis is the term applied to the vomiting of grossly visible blood. The blood may be bright red or darkened as a result of the conversion in the stomach of hemoglobin to hematin and other pigments by hydrochloric acid.

TABLE 6–1.   Estimation of Severity of Bleeding from Physical Findings

Sign	Approximate Reduction in Blood Volume (%)
Shock (hypotension, tachycardia, cold clammy skin)	
Recumbent	50
Orthostatic	20–30
Massive hematemesis	33–50
Pulse > 110 and systolic blood pressure < 100 mm Hg	30
Drop in blood pressure > 10 mm Hg and rise > 20 in pulse rate when raised from supine to sitting position	1 liter loss
Loss of color in palmar creases	50

Adapted from Schuster MM. Gastrointestinal hemorrhage: Stomach and duodenum. Curr Clin Digest 1966; 33(October):1551–1564.

Such darkened blood is frequently referred to as "coffee grounds." Bleeding from the upper gastrointestinal tract often leads to both hematemesis and melena (black, tarry stools containing altered blood) but either may occur alone. To observe melena in the absence of hematemesis is not unusual. Hematemesis almost always is a sign of bleeding into the esophagus, stomach, or duodenum, such as from a site proximal to the ligament of Treitz. Bright red blood in emesis typically points to a source proximal to the pylorus. Only rarely is hematemesis caused by bleeding into the small intestine.

---

*"**H**ematemesis almost always is a sign of bleeding into the esophagus, stomach, or duodenum."*

Illustrative Case

You are summoned to the emergency department to see a 67-year-old man who vomited bright red blood once, 1 hour before being admitted. The physician on emergency call has made a preliminary assessment and has started an intravenous infusion of normal saline. Orders have been issued for a complete blood count, prothrombin time, partial thromboplastin time, serum urea and creatinine, and typing and cross-matching for four units of packed red blood cells.

You learn that for the past 6 weeks the patient has had gnawing pain in the left epigastrium two or three times a day, appearing about an hour after meals. The patient said that milk and other foods relieve the pain. Pain has not extended beyond the epigastrium and has not awakened the patient during the night. You are told that the patient has been taking a diuretic agent for hypertension, ibuprofen 400 mg three times a day for arthritis, and a sedative at bedtime. He said that he imbibes alcohol only occasionally. One hour after entering the emergency department, the patient was observed to vomit 400 ml of bright red blood

The physician on duty is concerned because he is aware of how unpredict-able the course of patients with hematemesis can be. Guided by the volume of blood loss as estimated from the physical findings (see Table 6–1), sufficient packed cells are transfused to restore circulating blood volume. Concomitantly, the source of bleeding is sought, considering the possible causes listed in Table 6–2.

Comment. Serious bleeding results in hypovolemia, which is evident in the patient's appearance, cardiac rate, blood pressure, respiratory rate, and jugular venous pressure. The skin is assessed for color, clamminess, cyanosis,

TABLE 6–2.   Classification of Causes of Hematemesis

Diseases of the Alimentary Tract
  Diseases of the esophagus
    Esophagogastric varices
    Esophagitis
    Esophageal ulcer
    Mallory-Weiss syndrome
    Malignant and benign tumors
    Miscellaneous lesions
  Diseases of the stomach and duo-
    denum
    Chronic peptic ulcer
    "Stress" ulcerations
    Gastric erosions and gastritis
    Recurrent ("stomal") ulcer
    Malignant gastric neoplasm
    Benign tumors of the stomach
    Hiatus hernia
    Trauma
    Foreign bodies
    Prolapse of gastric mucosa into
     the duodenum
    Rupture of sclerotic vessel
    Gastric Diverticulum
    Specific infections
    Heteropic pancreatic tissue
    Miscellaneous gastric disorders
    Postoperative hemorrhage
    Duodenitis
    Duodenal diverticulum
    Duodenal tumors
  Diseases of the small intestine
Diseases of Neighboring Organs
  Swallowed blood
  Rupture of aneurysm, growth, or
   abscess
  Disease of the biliary tract:
   hemobilia
  Disease of the pancreas

Systemic and Organ System Diseases
  Amyloidosis
  Multiple myeloma
  Sarcoidosis
  Uremia
  Systemic infections
  Cardiac disease
  Ischemic gastrointestinal disease
  Pheochromocytoma
  Kaposi's sarcoma
  Collagen diseases
  Multiple neurofibromatosis
  X-ray–induced telangiectases of the
   bowel
  Miscellaneous disorders
  Diseases of the blood
    Polycythemia rubra vera
    Leukemia and lymphomas
    Pernicious anemia
    Thrombocytopenic purpura
    Nonthrombocytopenic purpura
     (allergic purpura, Henoch-
     Schönlein syndrome)
    Thrombocytopathy and thrombo-
     asthenia
    von Willebrand's disease
    Autoerythrocyte sensitization
    Hemophilia
    Christmas disease
    Hypoprothrombinemia
    Fibrinogenopenia
    Disseminated intravascular coagu-
     lation
  Diseases of blood vessels
    Hereditary hemorrhagic telangiec-
     tasia
     (Rendu-Osler-Weber disease)
    Pseudoxanthoma elasticum
     Grönblad-Strandberg syndrome)
    Diffuse vascular malformations
    Cavernous hemangiomatous mal-
     formations
     (blue rubber bleb nevus)
    Ehlers-Danlos disease
    Other rare vascular malformations

Modified from Berk JE, Haubrich WS, Kalser MH, Roth JLA, Schaffner F, eds. Bockus Gastroenterology. 4th ed. Philadelphia: WB Saunders, 1985:67.

and mottling. In patients whose hemoglobin is more than 50 percent of normal, hyperextending the fingers will usually cause the palmar creases to redden if they were previously pale (see Table 6–1). A systolic blood pressure lower than 100 mm Hg in a previously normotensive patient, with a heart rate exceeding 100 beats per minute, suggests a reduction of about 20 percent in circulating blood volume.

How serious is this patient's bleeding? Is it massive? Will he be one of about 20 percent of those with massive bleeding who will require surgical intervention? Many ill-defined terms are used to describe the grade and degree of hematemesis: massive, torrential, gross, severe, profuse, brisk, moderate, mild, minor, and trivial. No standard criteria have been established to delineate varying grades of bleeding. Such criteria are difficult to set, in part because the changes are dynamic and require repeated appraisal of clinical features and certain telltale laboratory determinations.

The terms "massive" and "severe" usually are applied to bleeding in the patient who is in hypovolemic shock with a hemoglobin concentration of less than 8 g per deciliter, a red blood cell count lower than 3 million per millimeter^3, and a blood volume 40 percent below normal. Approximately 20 percent of patients with hematemesis and melena will have bleeding severe enough to be designated massive or severe. Massive bleeding is unpredictable. It can become evident suddenly or gradually. What is initially considered as mild or moderate bleeding can become massive hemorrhage within minutes, hours, or any time later.

Clinical manifestations will depend upon the amount of blood loss, the rate of bleeding, and whether active bleeding ceases, persists, or recurs. Symptoms and signs also will be affected by the patient's previous hemodynamic status, together with the effects of bleeding on normal or abnormal cardiovascular, pulmonary, and renal systems. There is considerable variation, from patient to patient, in the amount of bleeding necessary to produce symptoms, shock, or death. The amount and rate of blood loss that can induce shock depends on numerous factors, including age, antecedent vigor or debility, and pre-existing anemia.

Estimates by the patient, a family member, or a friend in the amount of blood loss are often inaccurate. Similarly, assessment of blood loss based on the patient's initial appearance and presenting symptoms can be misleading.

Hematemesis of almost any degree is often accompanied by faintness, giddiness, weakness, chills, sweating, nausea, thirst, and anxiety. Even the occurrence of syncope does not necessarily mean there has been massive hemorrhage. Some persons tend to faint at the mere sight of blood. Conversely, collapse may be the initial manifestation of massive bleeding not yet evident by hematemesis or melena.

Because the plasma volume is quickly restored, gastrointestinal bleeding not exceeding 500 ml usually causes few symptoms. With more extensive bleeding and decreased circulating blood volume, there is a fall in venous return and cardiac output. Compensatory mechanisms, especially reflex vaso-constriction, are rapidly invoked to maintain effective blood supply to vital centers at the expense of less vital areas. Generalized vasoconstriction favors mobilization from blood reservoirs, marked by a shift of blood from the venous pool into the arterial portion of the circulation. Movement of extracellular and extravascular fluid into active circulation is another compensatory mechanism. The patient's antecedent state of hydration and cardiovascular status additionally affect the adequacy of compensatory mechanisms.

"Gastrointestinal bleeding not exceeding 500 ml usually causes few symptoms."

Hypovolemic shock, the major consequence of massive hemorrhage, occurs when the cardiac output is insufficient to fill the arterial tree with blood under sufficient pressure to provide adequate blood flow within vital organs and tissues. The net result is cellular hypoxia. Clinically, hypovolemic shock is characterized by a rapid, thready pulse and hypotension, with the systolic blood pressure below 80 mm Hg. If conscious, the patient complains of feeling cold and thirsty. Breathing may be rapid and shallow. Cerebral hypoxia causes restlessness, anxiety, and agitation. The skin, particularly of the extremities, is pallid, cool, and clammy. Light pressure on the skin induces blanching that is slow to change when pressure is relieved. Superficial veins, normally blue and distended, are collapsed and barely visible.

With uncorrected shock, respiratory difficulty increases and breathing becomes shallow and feeble. Prolonged shock and reflex vasoconstriction lead eventually to tissue anoxia and changes in the acid-base balance in the direction of metabolic acidosis. This is followed by a loss of arteriolar tone, collapse of peripheral resistance, further decrease in capillary blood flow, and ultimately to circulatory and myocardial failure.

The interval between impending and obvious clinical shock may be only minutes or as long as several hours. The systolic blood pressure may remain normal or even slightly elevated so long as reflex peripheral vasoconstriction is sufficiently maintained to compensate for reduction in cardiac output. This circumstance may persist for some time, particularly when bleeding is slow. Thus, the blood pressure alone may not be a reliable indicator of the amount or gravity of hemorrhage or of impending shock. This often is the case in younger patients because of their greater capacity for reflex vasoconstriction. The diastolic rather than the systolic pressure more accurately reflects a diminution in circulating blood volume. However, it should be borne in mind that previously hypertensive patients apparently maintain the diastolic pressure better than normotensive persons.

A reduction in blood volume and arterial blood pressure is associated with, or may be preceded by, tachycardia. However, the apical heart rate is often increased only slightly; indeed, initially it may be normal or even decreased. The apical rate also is influenced by rapid intravenous infusion and by anxiety. The pulse volume usually is reduced. In spite of the limitations noted, determinations of the apical rate, and especially of blood pressure, are of paramount importance in assessing the patient's response to massive bleeding, detecting continuing or repeated bleeding, determining the need for transfusions, and evaluating the response to therapy. The blood pressure and heart rate should be monitored continuously or taken every 15 to 30 minutes at first, and then later at hourly intervals until the patient's condition becomes stabilized. Continued or renewed bleeding may usher in severe shock. This impending catastrophe is recognized by a continuously dropping systolic blood pressure, increasing heart rate, weakening of peripheral pulses, and increasing pallor, coldness, and clamminess of the skin.

The tilt test provides a simple and fairly reliable measure of circulating blood volume and is useful in detecting impending shock (see Table 6–1). In this procedure the blood pressure and heart rate are recorded while the patient is supine; these recordings are then compared with the same measures taken while the patient is sitting upright. In the upright posture, an increase in heart rate of 20 beats per minute or more or a drop in systolic blood pressure of 20 mm Hg or more indicates hypovolemia.

"The heart rate and the systemic blood pressure should be monitored."

Monitoring the central venous pressure provides a reliable measure of venous return to the heart. It also serves as a useful guide to the need for transfusion. Urine output measured hourly provides an excellent index of renal perfusion, which is decreased during hypovolemic shock as a result of diversion of blood flow from the kidneys to the liver and brain. A drop in urine output below 0.5 ml per kg per hour is evidence of impaired renal blood flow. This, in turn, can lead to elevated serum urea nitrogen levels and, eventually, to oliguria and renal shutdown. Ordinarily, anuria attending shock is associated with a poor prognosis.

Pulmonary, cardiac, and cerebral changes may be extant before the occurrence of hematemesis, and worsening of these changes may present serious problems following hematemesis. Hematemesis in patients with cirrhosis may precipitate hepatic encephalopathy. Low-grade fever, although not a feature of hematemesis alone, is not unusual after hematemesis and melena from any cause.

Digital examination of the rectum is usually deferred while a patient is in shock, except when there is evidence of hypovolemia without obvious blood loss. Tarry black feces or bright or dark red blood may be found on the examining finger. The presence in the rectum of fresh or cherry-red blood suggests persistent or current bleeding. Also, rectal examination may disclose a Blumer's shelf, suggesting the possibility of metastatic neoplasm. In an anuric male patient, a large prostate may suggest bladder-neck obstruction as a cause rather than hypovolemia.

Further Information Pertaining to the Case.   While you are attending the patient in the emergency department, his vital signs remain stable; blood pressure is 110/70 and the apical heart rate is 90. The jugular venous pressure is decreased. The tilt test shows a postural drop of 15 mm Hg in the systolic blood pressure and an increase of 20 beats per minute. Monitoring the central venous pressure has been held in reserve for use if hematemesis recurs. Saline is being administered intravenously in both forearms, and 4 units of packed red blood cells are on their way from the blood bank. An H_2-receptor antagonist is being administered intravenously. The patient has been catheterized and has a good urine output. An electrocardiogram shows no abnormality. Fluid intake and output are being carefully charted. A nasogastric tube has not been inserted, as the patient is free of nausea and is able to take by mouth 30 ml of a nonabsorbable antacid every hour.

Further Comment.   In the presence of hypovolemic shock, active treatment is given promptly without extensive questioning or physical examination. In most cases, however, both history taking and physical examination can proceed concurrently with the institution of therapeutic measures.

The salient features of the patient's symptoms are elicited. Questioning a family member or friend may provide a clue to the cause of bleeding and can help clarify any medication the patient has been taking.

Is this the first time the patient has vomited blood? Or has there been evidence of gastrointestinal bleeding before? If so, when did this occur? How severe was the bleeding? Was hospitalization required? Were blood transfusions given? How many? And to what was the bleeding ascribed? Was the diagnosis established clinically, by radiography, or by endoscopy? Although important to note, a history of previous bleeding may or may not be helpful in considering the cause of the present episode of hematemesis. In as many as 25 percent of cases, a repeated episode of bleeding is from a source other than that found or postulated in a previous episode.

In consideration of peptic ulcer as a source of bleeding, it is known that antecedent ulcer pain is a feature in about 80 percent of patients. In most cases, this will be of the familiar pain–food–relief type (see Chapter 2, "Abdominal Pain"). One is reminded that the pain of peptic ulcer disease often is allayed by the onset of bleeding. In contrast, an absence of antecedent pain, along with signs of portal hypertension, favors the likelihood of bleeding from esophageal varices.

Examination of the abdomen is, of course, essential both in terms of positive and negative findings. In patients with bleeding ulcers, the abdominal examination usually is unrevealing, whereas the finding of a palpable mass or enlarged liver or spleen points in another direction. It is well to listen carefully to the abdomen of the patient who has had bleeding into the gastrointestinal tract. Loud, hyperactive bowel sounds suggest either an associated obstruction or the passage of a large volume of blood through the intestinal tract. A relatively quiet, soft, and nontender abdomen, on the other hand, can be somewhat reassuring in a patient who has bled.

"Pain of peptic ulcer disease is often allayed by the onset of bleeding."

Gastric or duodenal ulceration is high on the list of conditions that needs to be considered, because such lesions are common causes of hematemesis. In the case cited, the patient has taken ibuprofen, a nonsteroidal analgesic agent known to predispose to gastroduodenal mucosal injury and possible bleeding. The location of pain in the left epigastrium favors a gastric ulcer, as opposed to a bulbar or postbulbar duodenal ulcer.

The patient's long history of pain and the absence of acute, severe stress militates against so-called "stress ulceration" as the cause of hematemesis. In this or any patient of advanced age, gastric cancer would be considered, but this is a relatively infrequent cause of hematemesis. There was no antecedent history to suggest the esophagus as a source of massive bleeding.

Nothing was found on physical examination that would provide a clue to the cause of bleeding. Blood coming from another source, and then swallowed, was discounted because of the absence of any history of significant respiratory lesion and of any physical signs referable to the nose, throat, or lungs. Neither was a systemic hemorrhagic diathesis seriously considered. There were no mucocutaneous lesions, such as telangiectases. There was no purpura, lymphadenopathy, or splenomegaly that might suggest a blood dyscrasia.

There was no evidence of distended, readily visible, superficial, upper abdominal veins or caput medusae to indicate portal hypertension. There was no ascites, no venous hum over the umbilicus or arterial bruit over the liver that might suggest hepatic disease.

After thorough assessment of the symptoms and physical examination, a gastric or duodenal ulcer seemed the most likely source of hematemesis. Ibuprofen was strongly suspected of playing a role in contributing to the bleeding lesion.

Further Information Pertaining to the Case.   The patient was transferred to the gastroenterology unit. His condition remained stable, and he appeared comfortable. The hemoglobin level was nearly normal, possibly in part due to hemoconcentration from blood loss and incomplete restoration of total blood volume. Twelve hours after admission he was acutely stricken by nausea and again vomited an estimated 400 ml of red blood.

Comment.   In determining the course of treatment, the appropriate diagnostic procedure and level of intervention must be selected. When managing patients with hematemesis, consider the following:

- In as many as 80 percent of patients with hematemesis, bleeding stops spontaneously with conservative therapy. It is a matter of debate whether the diagnostic information obtained by upper gastrointestinal endoscopy provides a reliable basis for predicting which patients will stop bleeding and which will continue to bleed or will rebleed. One possible exception is the endoscopic finding of a visible vessel in a peptic ulcer crater.
- Medical management of hematemesis is much the same regardless of cause, except when bleeding is from esophageal varices. In the case at hand, there was no evidence of significant hepatic disease or its complications.
- Surgical intervention is required in about 20 percent of patients with massive hematemesis. The surgical mortality rate, especially in older patients who exhibit persistent or recurrent bleeding, begins to climb when operation is delayed more than 24 hours after the onset of bleeding. Surgical management is undertaken with greater assurance when the cause of bleeding has been determined preoperatively.
- The mortality rate in older patients with massive hematemesis, excluding that related to esophageal varices, is about 8 percent. Hematemesis due to gastric ulcer is more threatening than that arising from duodenal ulcer.

It became evident, because of repeated hematemesis despite supportive treatment, that surgical intervention would be required in this case. Among the diagnostic procedures that might be employed to help ascertain the site and cause of bleeding are air-contrast barium-meal radiography, esophagogastroduodenoscopy, radionuclide scintigraphy, and arteriography. Barium-meal radiography might have been considered if the patient had not rebled. Radionuclide scintigraphy might have demonstrated the site of bleeding but could not have revealed its cause. The major value of arteriography might have been in the expectation that simultaneous embolization to stop bleeding would be feasible.

Esophagogastroduodenoscopy was deemed the diagnostic procedure of choice for this patient. Many clinicians perform endoscopy as an emergency procedure in all patients with hematemesis as part of the so-called "vigorous diagnostic approach." Some physicians prefer to rely upon clinical judgment to decide when endoscopy should be done, believing that individualization in selection and performance of endoscopy is preferable to a rigid, ritualistic approach. All would agree, however, that endoscopy should be done when bleeding persists or recurs.

"Endoscopy should be done when bleeding persists or recurs."

Prompted by the course of events, and after having considered the options, upper gastrointestinal endoscopy was performed in this case. A chronic, actively bleeding ulcer situated on the lesser curve of the gastric antrum was seen. After adequate preparation, an antral gastrectomy with gastroduodenal anastomosis was done. The patient's recovery was uneventful.

Melena

Melena properly describes black, tarry stools containing altered blood. The resulting material, similar in color and consistency to tar, is glistening, coal-black, sticky, and exudes a foul odor distinct from that of ordinary feces. Melena derives from the hemoglobin of blood shed from the upper gastrointestinal tract, which in its passage through the bowel becomes darker red and eventually pitch-black. The color change is initiated by exposure to gastric acid. This can be evident at gastroscopy. Red blood oozing from an ulcerated lesion in the gastric mucosa turns dark brown almost immediately when exposed to the acid environment of the stomach lumen. The phenomenon is akin to a litmus test; shed blood that has been exposed to gastric juice and yet remains red is an indicator of achlorhydria. The degradation of hemoglobin to frank melena is furthered by enzymatic and bacterial action, given sufficient time, as shed blood traverses the lower bowel. Thus, the transformation of red blood to tarry stools is determined by the site of bleeding, the amount and rapidity of hemorrhage, the exposure of blood to acid, and the rate of intestinal transit. As a consequence of these factors, the most frequent source of bleeding that results in melena is proximal to the ligament of Treitz. It has been estimated that blood shed from a lesion distal to the duodenum must be retained in the intestinal tract about 8 hours in order to turn black, and probably longer to become tarry. The amount of blood required to produce a visible change in the stool depends on the level at which blood is shed. As little as 50 ml of blood introduced into an acid-secreting stomach can produce melena; as much as 250 ml of blood introduced at the cecum may be barely visible in the stools. This explains why patients who bleed relatively little from the stomach or duodenum sooner or later observe melena, whereas other patients may become severely anemic from blood loss in the colon and yet claim that they have never seen blood in their stools.

Blood shed in the alimentary tract, when present in any substantial amount, tends to exert a laxative effect. This is why patients sometimes describe the passage of melenic stools as "diarrhea." This also explains why large volumes of blood shed in the proximal gut may be rushed through the bowel, to the accompaniment of borborygmi, and evacuated while still red. Blood shed slowly and in small amounts does not have this effect and may be retained in the colon for an extended time, only to be passed as melena long after active bleeding has ceased. Tarry stools mixed with bright or dark red blood are sometimes passed together when bleeding from a site in the upper gastrointestinal tract is massive and the transit time is rapid.

"The most frequent source of bleeding resulting in melena is the area proximal to the ligament of Treitz."

Bleeding originating in the small bowel or lower may result in the appearance of black stools, but they tend to differ from the tarry stools of true melena in not being shiny or sticky. Moreover, often their surface has a dark red sheen, and when a fragment is placed on white absorbent paper there is a narrow red zone around the periphery of the stain. Such stools have been referred to as "pseudomelena."

Blood coming from the lower portion of the small bowel or ascending colon may have the appearance of dark currant jelly. When not profuse, such blood may be mixed with feces and be brownish black rather than dark red, particularly when passage through the colon is delayed. This also is apt to occur where there is obstruction at or beyond the bleeding site.

Not all red or black stools contain blood. It is well known, but still worthy of emphasis, that stools can absorb ingested pigments. Thus, a black stool may be noted after ingestion of compounds containing iron (e.g., hematinics) or bismuth (e.g., Pepto-Bismol) and foods containing charcoal (e.g., licorice). Although a distinction from true melena cannot always be made by the naked eye, stools darkened by iron tend to be greenish-black, whereas stools darkened by bismuth tend to be gunmetal gray. The thoughtful physician always reminds his or her patients of this phenomenon when prescribing medications containing iron or bismuth. Reddened feces may follow ingestion of beets in large quantities. Drug- or food-imparted coloration should be suspected when such stools are passed in the absence of obvious illness or other signs of blood loss. Confirmation, of course, is the negative reaction to tests for occult blood.

Illustrative Case

A 67-year-old man was brought by police ambulance to the emergency room because of increasingly frequent and copious melena over the preceding 6 days. He was well known, by virtue of numerous visits to the clinic and hospital, to the entire staff; only the admitting intern was making his acquaintance for the first time. Eight years earlier he had been admitted because of melena that was found to be due to bleeding from ruptured esophageal varices. Bleeding ceased with supportive therapy. Following recovery, a diagnosis of far-advanced alcoholic cirrhosis was established by liver biopsy. By surviving, the patient refuted what was thought to be a dire prognosis. He claimed to have given up his penchant for whisky, but the staff was never convinced that this was true.

Within a year the patient again was admitted because of melena, which was again found to be due to esophageal varices. Somewhat hesitantly, the staff recommended a shunt operation to alleviate portal venous hypertension. The patient sailed through the operation and convalescence with aplomb. He did not again show signs of bleeding. However, he did later exhibit intermittent hepatic encephalopathy for which a low-protein diet and neomycin were prescribed. It was uncertain that he adhered to his diet or took his medication. Almost annually this patient was the subject of a teaching conference; his initial liver biopsy slide would be reviewed, and everyone would marvel at his survival.

---

*"**B**leeding originating in the small bowel or lower may result in black stools."*

At this most recent admission, the patient was able to respond to simple questions by nodding or shaking his head, but he was hardly alert. His skin and sclerae were faintly icteric; his habitus was arachnoid. A tilt test, gently performed, indicated hypovolemia. While being prepared for admission to the hospital, the patient vomited a large volume of fresh and clotted blood. A specimen of blood was taken for blood counts and blood chemistries, and for type- and cross-matching; an intravenous infusion of saline was begun. Awaiting delivery of packed red blood cells from the blood bank, it was decided to perform emergency endoscopy following gastric lavage. Although aspiration through an Ewald tube yielded a good deal of blood, the endoscopist encountered much residual blood in the lower esophagus and stomach. This seriously hampered the endoscopic view. Varices were evident in the distal esophagus, but it could not be verified that bleeding was coming from the distended veins. The less than satisfactory endoscopic examination was terminated.

By this time, a unit of packed red blood cells was being infused into both arms. A Sengstaken-Blakemore tube was being readied for insertion with the hope that this might help stanch the flow of blood from esophageal varices. As the patient was being trundled to the intensive care unit, he soiled the gurney with an involuntary rectal expulsion of dark red blood, vomited fresh red blood, and expired.

Necropsy confirmed the presence of end-stage cirrhosis complicated by ascites, evidence of portal hypertension despite an apparently patent shunt, and extensive collateral venous channels. There were esophageal varices but no sign of erosion or perforation. In the fundus of the stomach there was a large, deep, scarred ulcer. In its base was the open knuckle of a medium-sized artery.

Comment.   This sad case with a turbulent ending conveys several messages pertinent to massive gastrointestinal hemorrhage. The first reiterates the point made earlier: recurrent bleeding can never be assumed to originate from the same source as that established as the cause of a previous episode. Here the setting compelled an assumption that massive hemorrhage probably issued from esophageal or gastric varices. If the Sengstaken-Blakemore tube had been inserted, it would have been to no avail.

> *"**R**ecurrent bleeding should not be assumed to originate from the same source as in a previous episode."*

The second message also reiterates a previous point: gastrointestinal bleeding is notoriously unpredictable. In this instance, a patient was admitted because of melena that had been noted for almost a week; yet during that time there was no sign that massive eruption of blood would be a terminal event. At admission the patient probably was more impaired by loss of blood than was appreciated; his obtuseness was attributed, perhaps mistakenly, to his previously observed hepatic encephalopathy.

A third point is that the benefit of endoscopy is only as good as the view obtained. To peer into a viscus awash with blood puts even the most perspicacious endoscopist at a disadvantage. Nevertheless, the chance of finding that the source of bleeding was a gastric ulcer and not an esophageal varix was within grasp but was missed. Arguably, as events precipitated, the finding might have made little difference in the eventual outcome. But if the gastric ulcer with a visible vessel had been recognized, active bleeding might have been stopped by endoscopically guided coagulation. In a precarious situation such as this, there are a good many "ifs" and little that is certain.

The clinical manifestations of hypovolemia and hypovolemic shock are the same whether caused by hematemesis or melena. Interestingly, the mortality rate of patients with melena alone is about one-half that of patients who present with hematemesis, and about three-quarters that when hematemesis and melena occur together. This is in part due to the fact that patients with hematemesis often include those who are bleeding from esophageal varices, a condition entailing high risk. Also, active bleeding that occurs during a patient's hospitalization is fraught with several times the mortality of that which occurs before admission to the hospital.

The diseases listed in Table 6–2 may, in fact, cause not just hematemesis but also concomitant hematemesis and melena, or melena alone. Although hematemesis by itself may be the presenting feature, melena often follows soon after or even a day or so later. When melena is the first manifestation of bleeding, subsequent hematemesis usually implies a severe exacerbation of hemorrhage and indicates a grave risk.

Bleeding from a chronic gastric ulcer is characterized by hematemesis more often than by melena alone, whereas bleeding from a chronic duodenal ulcer results in melena alone about twice as often as it causes hematemesis.

Gastrointestinal bleeding of any degree almost always entails an element of stress. In some cases the question arises: is stress the cause or the effect of bleeding? When a stressful circumstance can be recognized as occurring well before signs of bleeding, the possibility is entertained that stress may have induced gastrointestinal mucosal erosions that then bled. In such cases, there is usually no antecedent history of acid-peptic pain or distress.

Of what value is nasogastric intubation and aspiration? In the case presented here, the patient was intubated, but for the purpose of cleansing the stomach, not for diagnosis. In other instances, gastric aspiration can help to relieve nausea and vomiting that sometimes attend bleeding. Gastric aspiration for the purpose of diagnosis is superfluous in the patient who spontaneously vomits blood. In patients presenting with melena alone, a nasogastric tube can be useful in helping to identify the level of bleeding. A Levin-type tube is introduced slowly to the estimated level of the esophagogastric junction, about 40 cm from the incisor teeth. Water is injected into the tube and then gently aspirated with a syringe. If the aspirate contains blood, the bleeding site probably is in the esophagus or stomach. If no blood is evident, the tube is passed further into the stomach and aspiration is repeated. An absence of blood in the gastric aspirate, assuming bleeding is active, points to a bleeding site beyond the stomach. The procedure is simple, safe, and of diagnostic value if grossly visible blood is recovered. One is reminded that aspirates obtained in this manner should not be tested for occult blood. Insertion and manipulation of the nasogastric tube alone, in the absence of a bleeding lesion, is sufficient to produce a positive reaction for occult blood and, therefore, such a test will be misleading. It should be remembered, too, that in about 15 percent of patients with clear gastric aspirates, an actively bleeding lesion will be found by endoscopic examination.

Currently, barium-meal examination seldom plays a part in the search for a lesion producing upper gastrointestinal bleeding, its former role having been superseded by endoscopy. Not only is endoscopy more accurate in depicting mucosal surfaces, but the presence of clotted blood in the stomach can produce misleading defects in radiographically obtained images. Moreover, endoscopy, even though invasive, often requires less manipulation of the patient and, with portable equipment, can be performed at the hospital bedside. Finally, in selected cases, endoscopy provides an opportunity for therapeutic intervention by application of electrocoagulation or a heat probe to the bleeding site, or by injection of a vasoconstrictor substance or simple saline.

"In about 15 percent of patients with a clear gastric aspirate an actively bleeding lesion is found on endoscopy."

Bleeding from lesions in the small intestine can be variably manifest. Stools may be tarry or black, maroon or bright red, or mixed, depending on the bleeding site, the severity of hemorrhage, and the intestinal transit time. Bleeding from the small intestine accounts for about 3 percent of all cases of melena in adults. Among the causes are benign and malignant tumors, Crohn's disease, diverticula (Meckel or other types), focal ulceration (nonspecific or drug-induced), intussusception from any cause, angiodysplasia, and cirsoid aneurysms. Diagnosis is difficult insofar as available investigative procedures are limited. Advancement of a long intestinal tube seeking evidence of blood in serially aspirated material, supplemented by contrast radiography of areas yielding positive specimens, is a tedious and only occasionally successful maneuver. The most promising technique on the current scene is enteroscopy, using a specifically designed, thin, elongate endoscope.

Hematochezia

Hematochezia refers broadly to the passage of recognizable fresh or dark red blood from the anus. When bleeding originates from the distal colon, rectum, or anus, the blood is typically fresh and bright red. Blood originating in the ascending colon is more likely to be dark red. When the bleeding lesion is at or near the ileocecal junction, the fecal discharge may have a magenta hue and on standing is encircled by a ring of dark red blood, telltale characteristics to which attention was earlier directed.

If intestinal transit time is rapid and bleeding is brisk, dark or even bright red blood alone, or mixed with tarry or black stools, may be passed even though the bleeding site is located proximally in the gastrointestinal tract.

Illustrative Case

A 52-year-old woman has been passing red blood from the rectum for 12 days.

Clinical Assessment. The primary challenge is to try to determine which of the causes of hematochezia (Table 6–3) is most likely responsible for the bleeding as described and its probable site. To do this requires a series of pertinent questions and a few supplemental examinations, the choice of which is determined by the information obtained.

Duration and Frequency of Bleeding. Has rectal bleeding occurred before? Often patients tend to forget or overlook previous episodes, being preoccupied by the most recent occurrence. A history of previous bleeding, and how long ago it occurred, makes certain conditions more likely than others. Thus, for example, if the same sort of bleeding has been recurrent for a number of years, a malignant process is much less likely. In this patient, the recent episode of bleeding for 12 days was the first occurrence, and bleeding was observed during each of those days.

TABLE 6–3.   Causes of Hematochezia

Anal Canal
   Hemorrhoids
   Fissures
   Tumors
Rectum and Colon
   Colitis
      Idiopathic
         Ulcerative colitis
         Crohn's disease
      Infectious
      Antibiotic-induced
      Ischemic
      Radiation
   Tumors
      Malignant
      Benign
   Diverticulosis and diverticulitis
   Vascular malformations
   Other conditions
      Solitary ulcer
      Stercoral ulcer
      Traumatic ulcer
      Prolapse
Disease of the Small Intestine
Disease of the Upper Gastrointestinal Tract

Amount and Appearance of Blood Passed.   Is most of the blood on the toilet paper? Fresh blood streaking the toilet paper is frequently, but not necessarily, due to hemorrhoids or anal fissures. Is bleeding sufficient to redden the water in the toilet bowl? If so, this probably is blood that has dripped from the anus and is typical of bleeding from hemorrhoids. Fresh, fluid blood rapidly disperses in water, and only a few drops can turn the toilet bowl red. This explains why the patient often overestimates the volume of fresh blood loss. The passage of blood clots signifies more brisk bleeding. Seldom is fresh, anorectal bleeding sufficient to cause hypotension or hypovolemia, but it is possible. Abrupt, massive bleeding, usually self-limited, is typical of hemorrhage as a complication of diverticulosis or angiodysplasia of the colon. In this regard, it is well to remember that the presence of diverticula can never rightly be blamed for iron-deficiency anemia when there is occult blood in stools in the absence of intermittently brisk bleeding.

Is the blood bright or dark red? Bright red blood is more likely from anorectal and sigmoid colon lesions, whereas dark red blood is more likely from the more proximal colon.

> *"**B**right red blood passed by rectum is more likely to be from anorectal and sigmoid colon lesions; dark red blood from the more proximal colon."*

Relation of Blood to Bowel Movements.   What is the consistency of the stools? Are they hard and pellet-like? Does bowel movement require undue straining? Bleeding consequent to straining at stool tends to suggest the presence of hemorrhoids or anal fissures. Are stools soft and mushy? If so, they can hardly be the cause of anal abrasion. Is there urgency or incontinence? Has blood stained the undergarments? Bloody encopresis can be a sign of either hemorrhoids or anorectal neoplasm.

Has the patient been told of a previous diagnosis, such as diverticulosis, that might be responsible for bleeding? In a woman, is there a history of endometriosis?

Did constipation precede bleeding? The strained passage of hard stools may have aggravated hemorrhoids or produced anal fissures. Or has constipation followed bleeding? Because defecation is made painful by anal fissures, the patient dreads the prospect of bowel movement, tends to suppress the urge to stool, and thus aggravates constipation.

Red blood that streaks the surface of a stool is likely to originate in the anal canal or lower rectum, but bleeding from a proximal lesion may also coat a formed stool with blood. Small flecks of blood on formed stools that leach out red in the toilet bowl are typical of blood loss from polypoid lesions of the colon. Is blood intermixed with the stool? Distinguishing between blood *on* the stool and *in* the stool may have diagnostic importance; however, the average patient cannot be expected to provide accurate information on this point. When flecks of red blood are visible in the interstices of a stool, the bleeding lesion usually is in the sigmoid segment or rectum. When blood is thoroughly mixed within a firm stool, the source is usually proximal to the splenic flexure. These generalities do not apply, however, when the patient has diarrhea.

The passage of loose or liquid stools tinged with visible blood often signifies an actual enteritis with mucosal inflammation, erosion, or ulceration. But what the patient refers to as "diarrhea" may be rather a persistent feeling of urge to stool that is caused by a fecolith or rectal tumor. An unusual and peculiar form of mucoid diarrhea, sometimes tinged with blood, that can lead to electrolyte disturbance and even shock, is that due to exudation from a villous adenoma, usually situated in the rectum or sigmoid colon.

Further Information Pertaining to the Case.   On questioning, the patient states that she formerly had one formed bowel movement a day, but that for about a month before the onset of bleeding and since then she has passed 2 or 3 formed stools daily; that blood is passed with stools, but she cannot be sure whether blood is mixed or merely adherent to the stools. She denies any other bleeding tendency, and she has not been taking any form of anticoagulant medication. Her bowel movements have not been unduly strained or painful.

Further Comment.   Anal pain, during or after defecation, along with passage of visible blood, favors anorectal disease as the cause of bleeding. Such lesions include anal fissure, proctitis, and neoplasm. Pain is not a feature of internal hemorrhoids unless they are complicated by erosions, fissures, thrombosis, or anal stenosis. Intense pain that may be described as "tearing" or "burning" and that occurs during or immediately after defecation is a cardinal symptom of acute anal fissuring or thrombosed hemorrhoids; thereafter, pain lessens somewhat but persists. Severe throbbing pain, usually attended by fever and aggravated by bowel movement, is a feature of pararectal abscess, such as might complicate proctitis of any cause. Rectal or pelvic pain also is a feature of ischemic or radiation colitis.

Further Information Pertaining to the Case.   The patient describes mild, crampy, lower abdominal pain associated with urge to stool, then relieved by bowel movement. On recollection, the patient believes that this pain antedated her rectal bleeding by a month or longer. Pain has been intermittent, occurring 2 or 3 times a day, and lasting only a few minutes.

Further Comment.   Such pain suggests the possibility of a lesion partially obstructing the lower bowel. Neoplasm in the form of carcinoma would have to be high on the list of suspected lesions. Further questions would relate to the presence or absence of associated symptoms such as anorexia, change in diet habit, and weight loss.

"Anal pain during or after defecation, along with visible blood, indicates anorectal disease."

Further Information Pertaining to the Case.   Thorough physical examination was unrevealing of any clue to the cause of bleeding. With the patient on her left side, thighs flexed, and buttocks spread, the perianal area was examined for rash, fissures, fistulas, and signs of abscess; there were none. A few shriveled anal skin tags were evident, but there was no sign that these had bled. When the patient was asked to strain, there were no protruding hemorrhoids and no evidence of mucosal prolapse. No unusual tenderness was elicited as the examining finger was inserted in the anus. The rectal ampulla was of normal caliber and empty, save for a few small fragments of residual stool. No intrarectal mass or mucosal defect was palpated. No pararectal mass or tenderness was detected. With the examining finger fully inserted, the patient was asked again to "bear down." As the upper rectum and lowermost sigmoid colon came down to meet the finger tip, no abnormality was felt. When the gloved finger was withdrawn, a small fragment of feces was adherent and was seen to contain a faint streak of fresh blood.

Request was made for a complete blood count (looking for evidence of iron-deficiency anemia, leukocytosis, or platelet deficiency), urinalysis, and blood chemistry panel (to exclude the presence of unsuspected associated disease). In the light of the patient's history, it was decided not to order stool examination for ova and parasites or stool cultures. Because blood was plainly visible in the stools, it would have been fatuous to order tests for occult blood.

Meanwhile the patient was prepared for flexible proctosigmoidoscopy. This procedure confirmed the anal canal and rectum were clear. However, a thin trail of bloody mucus led into the sigmoid segment where, at the 35-cm level, a firm, nodular, circumferential, partially ulcerated lesion was encountered. The lesion so occluded the lumen that further passage of the endoscope was impossible. No biopsy was taken because the lesion obviously appeared to be a carcinoma that would require surgical segmental resection.

Further Comment.   The presumed cause of the patient's change in bowel habit, intermittently crampy abdominal pain, and rectal bleeding having been discovered, the patient was admitted to the hospital in preparation for the required surgical operation.

If the sigmoid lesion had permitted further advancement of an endoscope, complete colonoscopy would have been done to exclude the presence of another synchronous lesion proximally in the colon. Alternatively, a preliminary barium enema examination was considered for the same purpose; however, because the sigmoid segment was almost occluded by the neoplasm, it was believed that the risk of retained barium above the lesion outweighed the possible benefit of any information that might be obtained.

Further Information Pertaining to the Case.   Following a 3-day preparation of the bowel, operation was performed, consisting of anterior resection of the sigmoid segment with a primary anastomosis. The surgeon found no evidence of peritoneal or liver metastases. The resected specimen was found to contain a well-differentiated, circumferential adenocarcinoma that had penetrated all layers of the bowel wall but had not extended beyond the serosa; regional lymph nodes were slightly swollen and reactive but contained no metastatic carcinoma. The patient's postoperative course was uneventful.

Iron-Deficiency Anemia

There is yet another possible indication of gastrointestinal bleeding, more subtle than the visible expression of blood as discussed in the foregoing sections. This is the discovery of a hypochromic, microcytic anemia due to iron-deficiency that is presumably the result of blood loss, yet in the absence of overt hematemesis, melena, or hematochezia. There are numerous circumstances whereby a lack or loss of iron can result in anemia, however, in the temperate climes of the majority of developed countries, the most frequent cause is bleeding from the gastrointestinal tract.

If gastrointestinal blood loss has occurred and yet the patient is unaware of such bleeding, there can be only two explanations; (1) the amount of blood lost at any one time has been insufficient to be evident as hematemesis, melena, or hematochezia; or (2) the patient has not recognized blood as it appears in vomitus or stools.

As previously mentioned, a loss of at least 50 ml of blood from the upper gastrointestinal tract is required to produce melena, and a loss of as much as 250 ml of blood from near the ileocecal junction is required to change the appearance of stools. Iron-deficiency anemia can result from daily losses well below these volumes. It is not surprising, then, that a patient whose hiatus hernia oozes only 30 ml of blood daily will eventually become anemic; nor is it surprising that a patient whose cecal carcinoma exudes only 100 ml of blood daily will even more rapidly become anemic. Yet both patients will claim no visible change in stools.

What is surprising is the occasional patient found with a grossly bloody rectal mucosa who nevertheless denies hematochezia. One would think that because the color red is an almost universal signal of alarm or danger, a patient seeing red in stools would take note of the sign; however, failure to do so is not rare. Two possibilities may account for the error: either the patient has never really looked at the stools, or the patient is color-blind.

Occasionally a patient with iron-deficiency anemia may have observed melena but blamed black stools on something else: for example, "But I was taking iron at the time." Or the patient with hematochezia might say, "But I had beets for dinner one day." More probing questions can help correct such misapprehension.

It is beyond the scope of this chapter to explore the nuances of the diagnosis of iron-deficiency anemia. Suffice it to say here that iron-deficiency anemia often signifies gastrointestinal blood loss and that a patient's apparent unawareness of such loss can sometimes be dispelled by perspicacious questioning.

To Sum Up

Gastrointestinal bleeding is a common occurrence, appearing in various guises in every clinician's practice. Its guise can be penetrated and often its true nature identified by eliciting answers to properly selected questions put to the patient, supplemented by perceptive examination and appropriate tests. The three principal manifestations of gastrointestinal bleeding are hematemesis, melena, and hematochezia. Each of these can be analyzed according to data obtainable in the physician's office or at the patient's bedside. Early analysis of these potentially life-threatening manifestations may determine the patient's survival.

Suggested Reading

ASGE Publication No. 1009. The role of endoscopy in the patient with lower gastrointestinal bleeding. Guidelines for clinical application. Gastrointest Endosc 1988; 34(3) (Suppl):23S–25S.

Bogoch A. Bleeding. In: Berk JE, Haubrich WS, Kalser MH, Roth JLA, Schaffner F, eds. Bockus Gastroenterology. 4th ed. Philadelphia: WB Saunders, 1985:65–110.

Roth SH. Nonsteroidal anti-inflammatory drugs: Gastropathy, deaths, and medical practice. Ann Intern Med 1988; 109:353–354.

Leitman IM, Paull DE, Shires GT. Evaluation and management of massive lower gastrointestinal hemorrhage. Ann Surg 1989; 209:175–180.

Silverstein FE, Gilbert DA, Tedesco FJ, et al. The National ASGE survey on upper gastrointestinal bleeding. Parts I–III. Gastrointest Endosc 1981; 27:73–102.

Silverstein FE, Tytgat GNJ. Atlas of gastrointestinal endoscopy. Philadelphia: WB Saunders, 1987.

WEIGHT LOSS

William S. Haubrich, M.D.

7

The total body weight of an average adult comprises that of cellular protoplasm (about 50 percent), extracellular fluid (about 25 percent), adipose tissue (about 18 percent), and bone (about 7 percent). A notable change in body weight may reflect increases or decreases in any or all of these components. Although bone mass can and does change, its contribution to body weight is comparatively small and, therefore, can be discounted for practical purposes. Thus, when a person's total body weight increases or decreases, we are principally concerned with changes in the mass of protoplasm, the volume of extracellular fluid (both intra- and extracellular), and the mass of fat.

It is a marvel of metabolism that the average adult person's weight remains as constant as it usually does, from day to day and from year to year. There are minor fluctuations, to be sure, and some persons seem more liable to small changes—and more beset by them—than others. In some cases, minor fluctuations reflect altered patterns of eating or exercise; in other cases, fluctuations reflect intrinsic rhythms. Most of us, for example, undergo phasic variation in diuretic and antidiuretic activity. Many premenopausal women gain, and then lose, as much as several pounds of retained fluid before and after their cyclic menses. But these amount to relatively small changes in actual body weight.

What is abnormal, "clinically significant" weight change? Most clinicians would agree that any gain or loss exceeding 10 percent of a person's usual body weight is likely to signify a change that requires investigation and explanation. The degree of concern and the clinical significance depends, too, on the rate of change. A gradual, long-term gain or loss usually means a change in mass of protoplasm or fat; a more abrupt, short-term gain or loss usually reflects flux in fluid volume.

It should be kept in mind that all weight loss, especially that sustained by a previously heavy-set person, is not necessarily ominous or harmful. When adverse portents are absent, reduction in weight can lessen cardiac risk and diabetic diathesis.

How to Inquire About Weight Change

Note that "usual" for the individual person is not necessarily "normal" for the species. When assessing changes in weight of an individual patient in the office or at the beside, the physician is more concerned with that person's own customary weight than with national averages.

Actual weights, previous and current, should always be specified, thus enabling a quantitative comparison. It is not sufficient merely to record, "The patient has lost 20 pounds." Rather, it should be stated, "The patient now weighs 130 pounds, whereas 6 months ago the weight was 150 pounds." Expressing weight in comparative numbers allows for a quick calculation of percentage change. A 20-pound loss by a person who usually weighs 150 pounds (13.3 percent) is more significant than a 20-pound loss by a 250-pound person (8 percent).

It should be further clarified that the former 150 or 250 pounds was or was not the patient's usual weight. The inference differs according to whether the patient's customary weight was 150 pounds, or if the patient usually weighed 130 pounds, later gained to 150 pounds, and then lost 20 pounds, reverting to the usual weight.

The time span of weight change also should be carefully noted. Was weight lost within days or weeks, or did the change take place gradually, over a period of months or years? Moreover, the inference differs when the patient says, "It was three months ago I began losing weight, and I'm still going down," compared with, "A year ago I lost twenty pounds, but my weight hasn't changed now for the past nine months."

Often it may be difficult to be sure the numbers, if recalled, are accurate. It may be instructive to first ask, "Do you have a scale to weigh yourself at home?" or "When did you last weigh yourself?" Sometimes a patient may allege a certain gain or loss and yet be unable to verify a quantitative change in weight. There are other ways of approximating changes in body weight. One can ask a woman, "Has your dress size changed?" or ask a man, "Are you using a different notch in your belt?" Or one can ask either, "Do your usual garments fit more loosely?"

Further, one should know whether a change in weight has been a trend or a fluctuation. Once a woman announced to me that over the preceding 10 years she had lost 500 pounds. A startling statement! Of course, her weight when I saw her was the same as it had been a decade earlier. In the interval she had undertaken various schemes to lose weight, but in each instance she had been only temporarily successful.

Finally, often a patient may not have actually sustained the loss claimed. In a survey by Marton and colleagues of 1,200 consecutive patients, 8 percent alleged a loss of more than 5 pounds in the preceding 6 months. When the patients were carefully weighed, only half of these purported losses were verified. In my own experience, discrepancy between claimed and actual weight change is especially frequent among patients exhibiting an irritable bowel syndrome, in which true weight loss is seldom a feature.

"One should know whether a change in weight has been a trend or a fluctuation."

To What Does the Patient Attribute Weight Change?

Here the inquiry turns to the relation between weight change and concurrent or coincident circumstances. Of first importance is the patient's eating pattern. "Are you eating the same meals now as before your weight changed?" The answer may not be always reliable, but the response should be recorded. Patients can usually tell when their meals are smaller or less frequent. Asking patients to recount recent typical meals or better yet, if time permits, to keep a diet diary can be helpful in estimating relative caloric intake.

Not often is one confronted with "weight change of unknown origin." Of 91 patients found in the study by Marton and co-workers to have involuntarily lost an average of 26 pounds, a physical cause for the loss was evident in 59 patients (65 percent) and a contributing psychiatric disorder was apparent in eight (9 percent). Moreover, in most cases these clinicians were able to establish a valid physical cause following an initial, thorough appraisal. They later observed that an exhaustive search for inapparent disease was seldom productive in the long run.

Although cancer is the most frequently encountered physical cause of involuntary weight loss, other conditions to be considered include chronic infection, azotemia, and cardiorespiratory impairment. In any debilitating disease, body weight can decline as a result of increased basal metabolic activity, especially with fever of any degree and with accelerated catabolism. For a chronically ill person, even circumstances required for diagnostic and thera-peutic procedures, such as repeated or prolonged imposition of "nothing by mouth" or necessarily restricted diets, can take their toll.

If the patient has lost an appreciable amount of weight and yet is certain that appetite has remained vigorous, and if food consumption has been maintained or even increased, then the differential diagnosis is relatively simple: the patient has developed diabetes, or has become hypermetabolic because of an overactive thyroid gland, or has been unable to properly digest and absorb ingested nutrients. Associated symptoms are sufficiently evident, in most cases, to make the choice fairly easy. They include polyuria and polydipsia in the diabetic person; a stare, fine tremor, warmly moist skin, and tachycardia in the hyperthyroid patient (Fig. 7–1); and fatty and inordinately fetid stools passed

FIGURE 7-1.   This 31-year-old laborer, who prided himself on his physique, became alarmed when his weight plummeted from 195 to 110 pounds within only 2 months. During the same period, he had become extremely tremulous and had increasingly frequent, bloody stools. The cause proved to be the coincident onset of hyperthyroidism and idiopathic ulcerative colitis, an unusual but not unknown combination. At admission to the hospital, the patient's hyperthyroid state was evident in his "buggy-eyed" stare (A). When his thyroid gland and bowel were brought under control, he quickly regained 60 pounds (B).

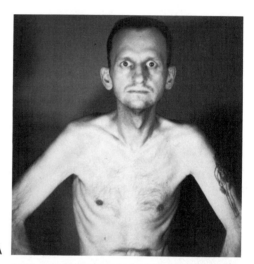

A

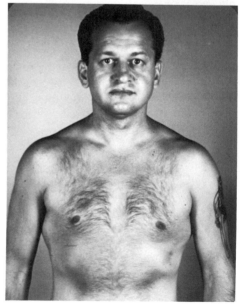

B

by the patient incapable of properly assimilating nutrients (Fig. 7–2). Among less-frequently encountered conditions in which weight declines while appetite and food intake seem preserved are certain leukemias and lymphomas, pheochromocytoma, carcinoid tumors, and infection by intestinal parasites.

> *"The patient may acknowledge a diminished food intake; the question is why."*

Commonly, however, the patient who has lost weight acknowledges a diminished intake of food. Usual meals are either skipped or only partially consumed. Again, the question is "Why?" Essentially, there are three main reasons why a person reduces his or her usual consumption of food (assuming food is available): (1) anorexia, (2) sitophobia, and (3) early satiety, listed in descend-

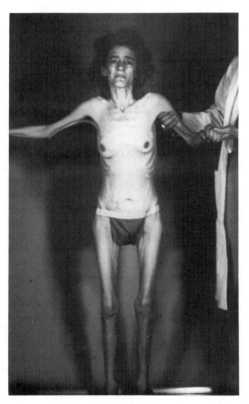

FIGURE 7–2. This 52-year-old woman was brought to the hospital because of progressive debility, her weight having dwindled from 130 to 75 pounds. Her chief complaint was that she no longer had the strength to rise from bed in order to obtain what had long been her daily ration of liquor. She had been remarkably free of pain but was troubled by a frequent urge to stool. Steatorrhea was abundantly evident. She died, despite treatment, a week after this picture was taken. At necropsy, her pancreas was found to be little more than a nodular, fibrous strand; her liver, interestingly, was entirely unscathed.

ing order of relative frequency (see Chapter 13, "Anorexia," and Chapter 14, "Eating Disorders").

Also to be considered are impaired sense of taste and smell, for any reason, or a painful mouth, such as plagues a person undergoing protracted dental procedures or burdened by ill-fitting dentures.

An indirect cause of weight loss of which the patient may not be aware is the influence of certain drugs or medications that he or she may be taking for an unrelated condition. For example, theophylline, commonly prescribed for asthmatics, often induces a queasiness that discourages eating. The taking of countless other drugs can be associated with overt or subliminal nausea and loss of appetite. In all cases, a complete record of recent medications is essential to a thorough assessment of weight loss.

"Acute weight change tends to reflect fluid flux; chronic weight change points to protoplasmic shifts."

How to Interpret Abrupt Changes in Weight

Acute variation in weight—up or down—usually reflects fluxes of body fluids, either retention or loss. Water is heavy; a liter weighs 2.2 pounds. Retention or dissipation of several liters or more of water is not unusual in certain circumstances and can account for considerable pain or loss in body weight. The flux can be in or out of either the intracellular or extracellular fluid compartments, or both. Shifts of extracellular fluid can involve the intravascular or extravascular spaces.

Dehydration, either by excessive loss of water or by insufficient intake of water, leads to a decline in body weight; added water, because of abnormal retention (sometimes due to excessive intake or administration of fluid), leads to a gain in body weight. Indeed, the simple procedure of weighing the patient at frequent intervals is an accurate means of assessing a flux of fluids. To ensure that comparisons are valid, it is important to see that the patient is being weighed at the same times from day to day.

Clinical signs of fluid loss, in addition to reduction in body weight, are pallor, poor skin and subcutaneous turgor (i.e., a pinch of loose skin in the forearm or back of the hand persists when the squeeze has been released), sunken eyes, collapsed superficial veins, orthostatic hypotension, and tachycardia. One does not have to make a patient stand up, and then watch him or her collapse, to demonstrate the peril of hypovolemia. Diminished circulating blood volume can be detected easily and reliably by the simple "tilt test" (see Chapter 6, "Gastrointestinal Bleeding"). Heart rate and blood pressure are recorded when the patient is quietly supine, and again after the patient has been raised to a sitting position. An increase in heart rate of more than 20 beats per minute, or a fall in systolic blood pressure of more than 20 mm Hg, indicates hypovolemia. A rise in heart rate is more significant and more easily counted.

One is reminded, in this regard, that lying flat in bed compensates for the effect of hypovolemia. When hypovolemia is suspected, it is not enough to ask the supine patient, "How do you feel?" The answer is likely to be "Fine." The same patient, put in an upright position, might complain of feeling faint and lightheaded. Hence, sit the patient up and then ask.

There is a special case in which very low plasma oncotic pressure leads to accumulation of interstitial fluid at the expense of circulating blood volume; the result is concomitant hypovolemia and anasarca, but the total body weight may be unchanged. Also, an apparently stable body weight can be misleading when observed in a cancer patient whose flesh has been wasted by inanition, yet whose pleural or peritoneal metastases have caused effusions of fluid in the chest or abdomen. Similarly, a patient with decompensated cirrhosis can develop a striking "arachnoid habitus" (spider-like appearance with spindly extremities and a ballooned belly) while body weight remains as usual.

Illustrative Case

A 68-year-old man, recently retired, sought a further medical opinion, hoping to elucidate the cause of a seemingly inexplicable decline in weight from his usual 165 pounds to 140 pounds, all in the preceding 6 weeks. He had been accustomed to generally good heath. Six weeks earlier he had been briefly hospitalized elsewhere because of an abrupt, intense, but evanescent abdominal pain. A single but significant peak elevation in serum amylase activity seemed to verify a diagnosis of acute pancreatitis. Severe pain dissipated after 24 hours of fasting supplemented by intravenous fluids. Later, oral cholecystography and upper gastrointestinal radiography were reported as normal. Back at home, the patient complained of only intermittent, relatively slight, upper abdominal soreness, although he found this irksome, as it interfered with his sleep at night. He was more concerned because of failure to regain appetite, inability to resume his usual eating habits, and his consequent loss of weight.

Physical examination disclosed the expected signs of substantial weight loss, but there was also a barely perceptible tinge of yellow to his sclerae and skin. When this was called to his attention, the patient recalled having observed the passage of unusually dark urine and pale stools. When specifically asked, he admitted to occasional itching. There was no abdominal tenderness or mass, no enlarged liver, and no accessible lymphadenopathy.

The laboratory reported bilirubin in the patient's amber urine, normal blood cell counts, slight elevation of serum bilirubin (5 mg per deciliter, predominantly in the "direct" or conjugated fraction), and elevated serum alkaline phosphatase activity (twice the upper limit of normal). Serum amylase and lipase determinations were in the normal ranges.

A chest radiograph showed clear lung fields and a normal heart silhouette. The only other procedure requested was a computed tomography scan of the abdomen. This disclosed a dense enlargement in the head of the pancreas and slight but definite distention of the common bile duct.

At operation, an unresectable carcinoma of the pancreatic head was found to be impinging on the common bile duct. There were several small metastases of carcinoma studding the surface of the right liver lobe. A choledochojejunostomy, using a Roux-en-Y construction, was done to restore egress of bile.

The jaundice and itching disappeared. Convalescence was uneventful; analgesics controlled the patient's pain. He did not regain appetite or weight, and within 5 months he was dead.

Comment.   The case of this unfortunate patient confirms several lessons. In older patients, acute pancreatitis (and this is doubtless what the patient had at the abrupt onset of symptoms), when attributable to no other cause, can be a herald of pancreatic carcinoma. This diagnosis must be considered in any older patient whose condition declines rather than improves following a bout of pancreatitis. In this case there was a strong suspicion of carcinoma, based on the clinical course alone, when the patient first sought further consultation because of weight loss. The need for surgical intervention was evident with a minimum of preliminary investigation. Operation, although not in any way curative, confirmed the diagnosis and conferred a measure of palliative relief.

To Sum Up

Variances from usual body weight can be indicative of the presence and evolution of disorder or disease. Abrupt loss of weight typically reflects dissipation of body fluids. More gradual or long-term loss of weight usually involves a change in cellular protoplasm and its constituents. Noteworthy is the degree of variation, relative to the patient's usual weight, and the span of time over which the change has occurred. Equally important are the circumstances in which weight loss has taken place. When all these factors are taken into account, an explanation of the change usually will become evident.

Suggested Reading

Bannister BE, Harvard CW. Patients who lose weight. [Editorial.] Br Med J 1983; 286:84.
Foster DW. Gain and loss in weight. In: Braunwald E, et al, eds. Harrison's principles of internal medicine. 18th ed. New York: McGraw-Hill, 1987.
Hall WD. Weight change. In: Walker HK, et al, eds. Clinical methods. Sec. 2. London: Butterworths, 1976.
Marton KI, Sox HC Jr, Krupp JR. Involuntary weight loss: Diagnostic and prognostic significance. Ann Intern Med 1981; 95:568–574.

DIARRHEA

G. Gordon McHardy, M.D.
William S. Haubrich, M.D.
J. Edward Berk, M.D., D.Sc.

8

Diarrhea, a near borrowing of the Greek word for "a flowing through," has been described in broad, simple terms as "the too-rapid evacuation of too-loose stools." For any given patient, however, what is called "diarrhea" depends, first of all, on the beholder. And the primary and principal beholder is, of course, the patient. As with constipation (see Chapter 9, "Constipation") no definition of the symptom can suffice, no matter how erudite the authority who presumes to define the term, until it is determined just what the patient means by diarrhea. The term is in common usage; everybody knows what it means, but in a given case no one knows what it means until the symptom is described by the patient.

Serious error can ensue if it is assumed that when the patient says, "I have diarrhea," the patient has passed profuse, watery stools; this may be the case, but the patient also may be referring to an unusually frequent urge to passage of formed stools. Or the patient may have had but a single urge to stool that day, but the passage was looser than usual.

What is thought to be diarrhea can depend, too, on the cultural setting in which the term is employed. A person habitually consuming a low-residue, omnivorous diet is accustomed to a once-daily, small, compact stool. Such an individual would likely call "diarrhea" the more frequent, bulky bowel evacuation of a person whose diet is mostly herbivorous.

An occasional patient may use the term *dysentery.* This, too, requires further description by the patient. The clinician may think of dysentery as being an intense urge to stool preceded by agonizing abdominal cramps; the patient may think of dysentery simply as passage of a loose stool.

Only for the pedantically inclined pathophysiologist is there a "correct" definition of diarrhea or dysentery. In the setting of the medical office or hospital, the definition is based on the clinical features in a particular patient so afflicted, and on the departures from that patient's customary stooling pattern. Thus, in the context of the simple definition of diarrhea previously noted, "too rapid evacuation" must take into consideration the variance in frequency normally experienced by a given patient. Similarly, "too loose stools" is meaningful only as it contrasts with the usual consistency of the patient's stools.

> "**W**hat the patient means by 'diarrhea' is fundamental to the definition and interpretation of the symptom."

Mechanisms of Diarrhea

A brief review of intestinal physiology and defecation can provide a basis on which to interpret a patient's complaint of diarrhea. A too-frequent passage of too-loose stools, to begin with this common concept, is actually the result of malabsorption of intestinal water and its congeners, arising from various alterations. Few people are aware of the tremendous flux of fluid in their bowels each day. About 10 liters (2 liters ingested, 1 liter of saliva, 2 liters of gastric juice, 1 liter of bile, 2 liters of pancreatic juice, and as much as 2 liters secreted by the intestine itself) enter the bowel in a 24-hour period; yet only a small fraction (no more than 0.1 to 0.2 liter) exits the bowel as fecal water (Fig. 8–1).

Nearly all the fluid entering the bowel is reabsorbed, so that the remnant of fluid and other components that together comprise the feces ultimately evacuated by the average normal adult on a Western-type diet weighs less than 200 grams, of which 60 percent to 80 percent is water. While the colon itself normally absorbs about 1 liter of water, it has a reserve capacity to absorb an additional 4 or 5 liters each day. Thus, even when the small intestine fails to absorb its normal share, the colon can accommodate the excess, up to a point.

What this means is that when the efficiency with which the intestine absorbs water is curtailed even slightly (reduced, for example, from 98 percent to 94 percent), the watery volume of daily stool output can be tripled. For most people, this would constitute annoying diarrhea. More serious impairment leading to still more voluminous stools can be alarming. It is not surprising,

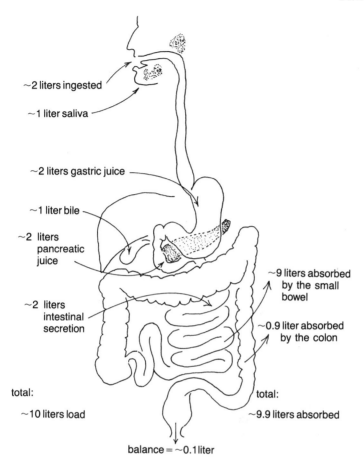

~2 liters ingested

~1 liter saliva

~2 liters gastric juice

~1 liter bile

~2 liters pancreatic juice

~9 liters absorbed by the small bowel

~0.9 liter absorbed by the colon

~2 liters intestinal secretion

total:

~10 liters load

total:

~9.9 liters absorbed

balance = ~0.1 liter

FIGURE 8-1. Normal fluid flux in the gut can be conveniently, if perhaps simplistically, thought of in terms of tens and tenths: 10 liters in from the mouth to the ileocecal junction, all but one-tenth absorbed by the small intestine, and a similar fraction of the remainder absorbed by the colon, leaving little more than one-tenth of one-tenth of the load as fecal water. Any appreciable excess of that small residual fraction is commonly called "diarrhea."

then, that any departure from normal in the direction of too-frequent passage of too-loose stools is a matter of consternation to the person so afflicted.

The daily stool weight of patients with diarrhea generally exceeds 200 grams and the water proportion is increased to as much as 90 percent. When the fluid content of the stools exceeds 0.3 liter per day, diarrhea is usually present.

What Can Be Learned from the Patient

Because such a broad array of information must be elicited, there is no recourse but to proceed with questioning in an orderly and thorough manner

(Table 8–1). Once the patient's initial definition of diarrhea has been obtained, the purpose of further questions is to seek an explanation of the problem in order to advise an appropriate remedy.

It is essential that a clear idea of the nature and character of the stools be obtained from the patient. Before questioning the patient on these points, however, it must be determined that he or she is in the habit of inspecting stool passages and, in particular, whether those of recent date have been observed. A description of stools is meaningless if the patient subsequently says, "But I can't bear to look in the toilet bowl after a bowel movement."

It should also be kept in mind when attempting to ferret out information that physicians since days of yore have used familiar substances as reference points in describing physical characteristics of tissues and various bodily excretions. Laypersons likewise tend to use well-known substances for comparison in describing expressions of ailments. It is of no great surprise, then, that a patient replying to a request for a verbal description of his or her stools will often express this best in similes such as "like thin porridge," "like dirty water," or "like coffee." Quite commonly, patients describe their stool passages as "watery." This description should be accepted with caution if there is no history of perianal soreness or evidence of perianal irritation. Most often, close inquiry will establish that the stools actually have some consistency and are not pure liquid.

To know the actual volume of stools would be advantageous, but the average patient cannot be expected to give a reliable estimate. Fecal fluid deposited in toilet bowl water cannot be measured. If the patient offers an estimate, it is almost always exaggerated. This is particularly true in cases of diarrhea associated with an irritable bowel syndrome. What the patient may claim to be "gallons of stools" turns out to be, if an actual 24-hour collection is made, little more than the normal half-pint.

Nevertheless, the average patient can readily distinguish between "large-stool" and "small-stool" diarrhea, and this can be an important distinction.

> "*It* is of value to distinguish between 'large-stool' and 'small-stool' diarrhea."

Stools described by the patient as being voluminous are usually abundantly fluid and indicate impairment of water resorption proximally in the bowel. Stools described as small "squirts" are usually mucoid in consistency and indicate anorectal irritability. For example, frequent urge to stool but with expulsion of only a pittance of substance is typical of proctitis with sparing of the proximal colon. The same sequence may be described by patients harboring rectal tumors. Occasionally, one may encounter a fastidious patient who

TABLE 8–1.   Questions to Ask When Interrogating a Patient with Diarrhea

1. Was the onset recent and acute? If so:
   (a) Were you out of the country recently or just before the onset? Did you experience diarrhea where you were?
   (b) Did you eat at a restaurant with which you were not familiar? Did you eat any food unusual for you, including raw meat, raw fish, raw or undercooked shellfish, raw milk, stream or well water?
   (c) Were others who ate with you affected?
   (d) Have you any pets at home that are ill?
   (e) Have you taken any medications that are new and not previously prescribed, especially antibiotics?
   (f) Are the passages explosive? Are they attended by abdominal pain?
   (g) Is the diarrhea associated with other symptoms (fever, nausea, vomiting)?
2. Is the diarrhea longstanding? If so:
   (a) For how long a period of time?
   (b) Is it intermittent?
   (c) Is it followed by periods of constipation?
   (d) Do the recurrences—if any—have any relation to emotional stress or strain?
   (e) Have you lost weight, become weak, or noted other symptoms?
   (f) Have you been in the habit of regularly taking some medicine over a period of time to ensure a daily bowel passage?
   (g) Have you undergone any operation on your stomach or intestines?
   (h) Has your diet changed? Are you ingesting more vegetables, soft drinks, or low-calorie foods?
3. What are the characteristics of the discharges?
   (a) Frequency?
   (b) Consistency?
       (1) If described as "watery," are they associated with perianal tenderness and soreness?
       (2) Similar in consistency to cooked oatmeal? or applesauce? or sausage?
   (c) Size and volume?
   (d) Can you recognize any food in the stool that you had eaten within the previous 24 hours?
   (e) Does the stool tend to stick to the toilet bowl and be difficult to flush?
   (f) Is it malodorous?
   (g) Does it appear foamy?
   (h) Does it float?
   (i) Are there any oil droplets?
   (j) Is there any pus or mucus on or around or mixed with the discharge?
   (k) Is there any visible blood?
4. Have there been any accidental discharges?
5. Are you awakened from sleep at night by the need to have a stool passage?

complains of "diarrhea," yet actually describes urgency, not to expel feces but rather to merely pass flatus.

Another point of distinction that should seem obvious, but may not always be evident until the patient is carefully questioned, is the matter of *encopresis*. This is a highfalutin term for involuntary fecal seepage from the bowel, such as often occurs in patients with incompetent anorectal sphincters. In some cases, the complaint is annoyance or embarrassment at repeated soiling of under-garments.

The patient may come closer to fact in describing the color of stools. Of chief concern is the presence of blood. One can ask, "Did you see any blood in your stools?" but then one has to inquire further "Was it pink, like currant jelly, bright red, maroon, or jet black?" Some patients become alarmed when they pass loose stools that are "awfully dark." For such occasions it is helpful to keep at hand a chart of painter's stains, available at any hardware store. The patient is shown the chart and asked to compare the sample chips with the observed color of stools. More often than not the "awfully dark" color is matched to that of a brown walnut stain rather than with the almost-black of deep mahogany. Obviously there are other pitfalls in attempting to determine the color of stools (see Chapter 6, "Gastrointestinal Bleeding").

One can check for occult blood in a specimen of stool from a patient complaining of diarrhea, of course, but the reaction can be misleadingly positive, especially if the specimen was collected on a gloved finger following vigorous rectal examination. Also, a patient who has undergone the rigors of frequent, forcefully expelled stools often will have superficial abrasion of the anorectal mucosa, allowing escape of enough blood to yield a positive reaction when chemically tested.

To ask if pus was seen in stools is futile. Rarely is purulent exudate so abundant as to be clearly visible, and hardly ever would it be clearly identified by the patient. (The presence of abundant white blood cells in a diarrheal stool is, of course, important, but this is a microscopic determination.)

"The more watery a diarrheal stool, the less likely it is to be fetid."

Even the presence of mucus, which is of less importance, is difficult to identify. Usually mucus is so mixed with water in a liquid stool as to escape detection. An exception is the diarrhea complained of by the patient whose frequent urge to stool is met with excretion of almost pure, ropy mucus; such a patient may harbor in the rectum or colon a mucus-secreting villous adenoma. Occasionally, a person may bring in a jar containing a congealed strand of mucus mistakenly thought to be an expressed worm.

The more watery a diarrheal stool, the less likely it will be fetid. This is because of dilution of odoriferous substances that may be present. When stench of loose stools is a patient's complaint, one thinks of steatorrhea due to intestinal malabsorption. (Steatorrheic stools of pancreatic exocrine insuffi-ciency are less fetid because undigested fat remains largely as triglyceride rather than being broken down to volatile fatty acids.) True steatorrhea of significant degree, such as may be reported as diarrhea in celiac disease, seldom escapes detection if the stool is actually observed and smelled. The most striking feature is the extremely fetid odor. To this point, one can ask if a deodorant such as "Air-Wick" is kept in the bathroom. Once a patient of mine answered, "Yes, at least a dozen." Another patient with unusually fetid stools had been forbidden by other members of his household to use the family bathroom; he was obliged to answer his urge to stool in the rest room of the corner gasoline station.

Usually, steatorrheic stools are pale in color, bulky, and mushy to soft in consistency, but they can vary from watery to cheesy; their volume, in a 24-hour collection, exceeds normal, sometimes considerably.

> **"W**hen inquiring about steatorrhea, ask if oil droplets have been noted."

When inquiring of steatorrhea, one should ask if fat or oil has been apparent in or on stools, and whether oil droplets, resembling drippings from the oil case of an automobile, has been seen floating on the water of the toilet bowl. With respect to such droplets, however, one should keep in mind that visible oil, unmiscible with water in the toilet bowl, is evident only when neutral fats are present (i.e., as in pancreatic steatorrhea). The visible fat in such cases tends to appear as pools of yellow or orange oil, because vegetable carotene is highly soluble in fat. Patients often are asked, "Do your stools float?" This is not a really perceptive question. Because most loose, fragmented, diarrheal stools will float in the toilet bowl water, this observation is not distinctive of steatorrhea. Stools more often float because of entrapped gas than because of excessive fat content.

The pattern of stooling should be carefully recorded. This includes notation of onset, duration, intermittency, and frequency. Abrupt onset suggests a precipitous cause, such as acute infection, toxin ingestion, vascular catastrophe, and fistula formation. Diarrhea of only a week's duration or less indicates an acute condition; diarrhea persisting for months or years is clearly chronic. Diarrhea that comes and goes with extended intervals of normal bowel action prompts a search for an intermittent precipitant. Alternate periods of diarrhea and constipation with seldom a respite of "normal movements" strongly suggests an irritable bowel syndrome.

A consistent diurnal pattern can be enlightening. It has been said that the urge to stool awakening a patient during the night indicates an "organic" cause as opposed to a "functional" disturbance. This is often, but not always, true.

Surely, diarrhea that persists both day and night points to a more serious disorder, but there are some patients with keenly irritable bowels who are troubled occasionally by nocturnal diarrhea. A pattern of short "runs" of diarrhea in the morning after breakfast and in the evening after supper, with respite during midday, is typical of an irritable bowel, but the same pattern is sometimes seen in patients with chronic idiopathic inflammatory bowel disease.

Frequency of bowel movement is easier to tabulate than volume of stool is to estimate. One can ask, "How many times did you move your bowels yesterday?" but the answer, if one is forthcoming, may not be accurate. Only an exceptionally compulsive person actually counts the number of trips to the commode. Another tack is to ask about the interval between urges to stool. Answers such as "every few minutes" tend to exaggerate frequency. It is better to construct a diurnal time line similar to that used to chart recurrences of abdominal pain (see Fig. 2–4 in Chapter 2, "Abdominal Pain"). If time permits (and this can be especially helpful when assessing chronic diarrhea), ask the patient to keep a "stool diary," carefully noting the time, consistency, and approximate volume of each stool passed, along with the time of eating, the content of meals, and other coincident circumstances. Such a diary not only may yield clues to the cause of diarrhea but also can be a helpful guide to later advising the patient of the most effective schedule for taking anticipatory doses of antidiarrheal medication.

> *"Nocturnal diarrhea points strongly, but not with absolute certainty, to an 'organic' cause."*

Chronic, persistent diarrhea, in the absence of other symptoms that might point to a cause, often is the most difficult to explain. If the patient is an elderly woman, consideration should be given to the possibility of microscopic colitis or collagenous colitis. It has not yet been determined whether these are related conditions. Neither condition is betrayed by specific symptoms, and the only basis for suspicion is chronicity, advanced age, and female gender. Colonoscopy is unrevealing of any mucosal defect, so that diagnosis rests on random mucosal biopsy.

Much has been made in the past of another condition characterized by chronic persistent diarrhea and also seen principally in older persons. This ailment, termed "gastrogenous diarrhea," was presumed to be related in some manner to gastric achlorhydria. Although the entity is controversial, it might not be amiss to consider achlorhydria as a possible contributor in an older patient who complains of the persistent passage of large, soft stools during the morning and after meals, for which no explanation is apparent.

Associated symptoms can give helpful clues to the cause of diarrhea. Of immediate importance in cases of acute or severe diarrhea are symptoms indicative of excessive fluid loss, dehydration, and consequent hypovolemia, such as compelling thirst, dry mouth, and orthostatic hypotension (for more on these symptoms and a description of the tilt test, see Chapter 7, "Weight Loss").

> "**D**iarrhea due solely to impaired fluid flux is usually painless."

Pain, or distress akin to pain, may or may not attend diarrhea. Diarrhea due solely to impaired fluid flux is usually painless; that caused by intestinal inflammation or hypermotility is often painful. Pain associated with diarrhea can range from intense, colicky cramps to anorectal soreness. Some patients, if questioning has been only cursory, fail to distinguish between pain and nausea or queasiness, the latter being frequently concomitant with diarrhea. Accompanying nausea, especially when attended by vomiting or retching, usually indicates irritation along the entire length of the alimentary tract, such as occurs in common and acute gastroenteritis. The latter condition is often referred to by patients as "intestinal flu" or "the crud."

The presence or absence of fever can be a key point. High, spiking fevers, particularly when attended by shaking chills, implicate acute infection and often bacteremia, viremia, or septicemia. Erratic fever of moderate degree suggests idiopathic inflammatory bowel disease. Low-grade fever can accompany dehydration due to any cause.

Weight loss coincident with acute diarrhea indicates dehydration. More gradual decline in weight associated with chronic diarrhea suggests underlying inflammatory bowel disease, neoplasm, or malabsorption. Chronic diarrhea as a manifestation of functional bowel disorder is almost never accompanied by weight loss.

Other telltale symptoms include skin rashes and flushes. Certain specific infections causing diarrhea, such as typhoid fever, can be identified by distinctive rashes. Intermittent flushing of the skin can betray humoral discharges, as in the carcinoid syndrome.

Circumstances attending diarrhea, whether or not they seem related directly to the alimentary tract, should be the subject of systematic questioning and, if present, duly noted. In cases of acute diarrhea, query is made about possible exposure to contagious disease. "Have other members of your family been similarly affected?" If diarrhea followed a shared dinner or public gathering, the inquiry would be "Do you know if others came down with the same trouble?" The answer may have epidemiologic implications.

If tainted food is suspected, the interval between ingestion and adverse reaction helps to distinguish the cause. Gastrointestinal upset and diarrhea occurring within a very short time indicates a reaction to a preformed toxin in poorly preserved food, such as that produced by staphylococci. Diarrhea occurring only after a number of hours suggests a toxic effect resulting from proliferation of pathogenic microorganisms within the gut lumen. A warning here: be cautiously circumspect in confirming a patient's suspicion of tainted food until or unless the evidence is compelling. Some persons are quick to blame acute diarrhea on supposedly contaminated food, especially that served in a public place. If such purported blame comes up in conversation, the prudent physician reserves judgment. Too hasty agreement with a patient's accusation may later lead to ill-founded litigation.

Included in liability to diarrheal disease might be recent travel—exotic and not so exotic. There are sensitive persons for whom even a weekend not far from home can disrupt bowel habits. The most familiar diarrheal affliction of travel is the common *turista,* usually associated with excursions by persons residing in temperate zones to more tropical climes. Here again, timing can be a clue. Turista typically strikes abruptly, but only after several days into the trip, and is usually self-limited after another few, sometimes agonizing, days. Diarrhea caused by protozoal infection, as by pathogenic amebas, does not appear until after an incubation period of about 2 weeks. Still more subtle and delayed can be the onset of diarrhea due to *Giardia* infection. In these cases, the locale of travel may help to identify the infection. Typical is the case of the hapless adventurer who kneels by a mountain rivulet, sipping the refreshingly clear, cold water, unaware that upstream there is a beaver dam whose denizens are loaded with *Giardia.* The diarrhea of tropical sprue rarely becomes evident until after many months or years of residence in an area where the condition is endemic.

Seeming emotional precipitants of diarrhea are more difficult to assess properly but should be considered. Surely they are common, but there is not always a temporal cause-and-effect sequence of proof. (One is mindful of the *"Post hoc, ergo propter hoc"* fallacy.)

The lifestyles of patients complaining of diarrhea must be taken into account. Opportunistic enteric infections are distressingly frequent in persons whose immunity has been impaired by acquired immunodeficiency syndrome (AIDS). Acutely annoying anorectal irritability and urgency to stool are typical symptoms of gonorrheal proctitis. Aerobic exercise has been known to induce "runner's diarrhea."

Inquiry should be made about diet, use of drugs, or exposure to potential chemical toxins, all of which can be related to diarrhea. The usefulness of a patient's diet diary has been previously discussed. Most lactase-deficient persons know from personal experience that they are prone to develop distressing symptoms, including diarrhea, after consuming milk and certain dairy products, although sometimes their memory has to be jogged. In contrast, persons whose "diarrhea" is actually the steatorrhea of celiac disease rarely associate gluten-containing foods with their bowel problem until their attention is called to it.

"Enteric infections are frequent in patients with AIDS."

Recollection of what has been ingested must include not only what was eaten at mealtimes but also what was consumed between meals. Some persons consume, but fail to mention unless specifically asked, prodigious volumes of so-called diet beverages. These may contain sufficient fructose to induce osmotic diarrhea. Imbibing alcoholic beverages in any quantity is well known to induce diarrhea in susceptible persons. Persons intent on losing weight commonly resort to "sugarless" foods, including chewing gum, and thereby consume large amounts of sorbitol. This substance is poorly absorbed in the small intestine and, on reaching the colon, is acted on by bacteria to form products conducive to diarrhea. Overweight persons also may take laxative agents in a misguided effort to shed a few pounds. Laxative abuse may similarly be a clinical feature in patients with an eating disorder (see Chapter 14, "Eating Disorders").

It is of utmost importance to inquire whether and how the patient's diarrhea has been altered during periods of fasting. Many patients with chronic or recurrent diarrhea have experimented with fasting at one time or another, and they will be prepared to answer the question. A patient may say, "When I don't eat, I'm OK, but as soon as I try to put something in my stomach, the diarrhea comes back." This is a strong indication of osmotic diarrhea. Another patient may say, "I've tried going without food for several days, but my diarrhea was as bad or worse than ever." Such a reply points to a secretory or "driven" diarrhea. The ultimate test of a relation of diarrhea to diet is to hospitalize the patient, carefully collect and measure the volume of stool expelled over a 24-hour period and then withhold all fluid and food by mouth (sustaining the patient by intravenous infusion), and repeat stool collections for another 48 or 72 hours. In cases of osmotic diarrhea, there is a dramatic decline in stool output; in cases of secretory diarrhea, the output is unchanged.

The list of medications, either prescribed or obtained over the counter, whose possible side effects include diarrhea is almost endless. Often the offending medication has been taken for a condition entirely unrelated to the digestive tract. Common examples are various cardiac agents (e.g., digitalis, quinidine), numerous antibiotic agents, nonabsorbable antacids, and colchicine. Lactose and lactulose are excipients in a number of pharmaceutical preparations and may be unknowingly consumed in sufficient quantity to induce diarrhea. It is important, therefore, to inquire whether new medication of any sort, not previously prescribed, has been taken.

---

*"**F**asting reduces stool volume in osmotic diarrhea, but not in secretory diarrhea."*

Allied to the role of medications and other iatrogenic factors in diarrhea is probing the patient's previous medical history. An example is the effect of autonomic neuropathy that can become evident in longstanding diabetes. Previously undertaken surgical procedures may be implicated. A fairly common example is a tendency to diarrhea in persons having had cholecystectomy; in such cases, the addition of gastric resection or pyloroplasty is almost sure to be followed by diarrhea. X-radiation therapy directed to the abdomen or pelvis can be a cause of diarrhea. The occurrence is bimodal (i.e., diarrhea may be evident during or shortly after the course of therapy), or an actual radiation enteritis may not be evident until many months following treatment. Intensely annoying can be the anorectal urgency, often described as "diarrhea," induced by radiation therapy adversely affecting contents of the pelvis. Chemotherapy utilizing potent cytotoxic agents can suppress immunity so as to render the patient susceptible to opportunistic bowel infection that often is manifested as diarrhea.

Particularly nettlesome is a suspicion of factitial diarrhea induced by the surreptitious consumption of laxative or cathartic agents. This information is never volunteered at the initial interview and seldom can be extracted later, even when the patient is confronted by incontrovertible evidence. These victims of their own misguided action often are not apprehended until they have induced severe dehydration and hypokalemia. The clinical presentation in such a condition is similar to that of a patient with severe secretory diarrhea. Surreptitious use of certain laxatives may be unmasked by chemical testing of feces or urine or by the finding of telltale changes in the colorectal mucosa. Thus, the development of a red or purple color in feces or urine after the addition of sodium hydroxide indicates the presence of phenolphthalein-containing drugs; the detection of melanosis coli at proctosigmoidoscopy signifies long use of anthraquinone cathartics.

Some Useful Test Procedures

Further insight into the nature of symptomatic diarrhea can be provided by a few relatively simple tests. Among them, the following are worthy of note:

1. Look at an actual specimen of the patient's stool. The appearance may be at variance with what the patient has described.
2. Arrange for a collection of all feces passed during a period of 24 hours or longer; measure the volume and weight. This, too, may be at variance with the patient's claim.
3. Examine a sample of feces under the microscope; look for white blood cells (indicative of mucosal injury, as with microbial invasion), red blood cells, parasites and their ova, fat, and undigested meat fibers.
4. Determine the osmolality of fecal fluid (normal osmolality = 336–423 milliosmol; diarrheal osmolality = 285–330 milliosmol; when osmolality of fresh stool samples is compared with 2(serum Na^+ + serum K^+), a negative osmotic gap commonly is associated with secretory diarrhea, whereas a high osmotic gap (>160 milliosmol) occurs with osmotic diarrhea.
5. Culture the stools. Bacteria may be absent when white blood cells are present, and vice versa.
6. Determine intestinal transit time by recording the interval between ingestion of a nonabsorbable marker such as charcoal and the appearance of black stools; or check the number and location of ingested radiopaque markers in serial plain films of the abdomen.
7. Test the effect of fasting on the frequency of bowel movements and the fecal volume. This is the simplest and most reliable means of distinguishing between osmotic and secretory diarrhea.

Illustrative Case

A 71-year-old woman consulted her internist because of several months of annoying diarrhea that had defied diagnosis and symptomatic therapy. She said that she daily passed from four to as many as 15 soft to watery, sometimes foamy stools that tended to float in the toilet bowl. Stools were frequent but, according to the patient, not voluminous. Defecation was attended by much flatulence, but other than urgency to stool, she had little or no abdominal distress. Her usual night's sleep had not been disturbed. Her weight had declined from 140 to 127 pounds.

Previous to the recent diarrhea, the patient had been bothered occasionally by constipation, which was corrected by the use of mild laxatives. Recent prescriptions for the diarrhea had included Pepto-Bismol, diphenoxylate, and loperamide, as well as several courses of tetracycline, sulfasalazine, and metronidazole, all to no avail. To allay mild arthritic pains, the patient occasionally took nonsteroidal, anti-inflammatory drugs in small doses with no apparent adverse effect. Thyroidectomy 10 years earlier necessitated hormone replacement therapy to achieve a euthyroid status. The physical examination was entirely unremarkable. The patient was subjected to extensive laboratory, radiographic, and endoscopic examinations, all of which were unrevealing.

The patient was then directed to a dietitian with a view to establishing a wholesome mealtime schedule. The dietitian issued strict and explicit instructions about what the patient was and was not to consume. She adhered faithfully to this instruction. Behold: the diarrhea disappeared, and the patient rejoiced in the resumption of a normal, satisfying bowel action.

Comment. The explanation of this happy although unexpected turn of events lay in elements of the history that had not been adequately pursued. It seemed that the patient was a travel agent who, because of long hours spent in her office, had consumed an inordinate amount of coffee. In recent months, because of a desire to reduce weight, the patient had added a nearly equal volume of "diet drinks," which she supplemented with "diet foods" devoid of sugar but rich in sorbitol. This provoked an osmotic diarrhea that subsided when the patient understood the more sensible regimen advised by the dietitian. The patient was well pleased with the outcome.

To Sum Up

Diarrhea is a common symptom that, despite its being an almost universal experience, always requires definition according to the concept of the individual patient. The vagaries of diarrhea have to be explored beyond the usual concept of "too-frequent passage of too-loose stools." In addition to eliciting a description of the symptom and the stool produced thereby, inquiry is properly directed to circumstances preceding or accompanying diarrhea. The reward of such meticulous inquiry is to arrive at an explanation of the disorder and establish its cause, which likely to lead to a remedy. What the late Francis W. Palfrey proclaimed over a half-century ago remains true: "Still, for the sake of happiness and efficiency, if not to save life, regularity of the bowels is a satisfaction which justifies earnest effort toward its attainment."

Suggested Reading

Blaser MJ. Infectious diarrheas: Acute, chronic, and iatrogenic. [Editorial] Ann Intern Med 1986; 105:785–787.
Debongie JC, Phillips SF. Capacity of the human colon to absorb fluid. Gastroenterology 1978; 74:698–703.
Field M, Rao MC, Chang EB. Intestinal electrolyte transport in diarrheal disease. N Engl J Med 1989; 321:800–806.

Phillips SF. Diarrhea—a broad perspective. Viewpoints Digest Dis 1975; 7(5).

Read NW, Krejs GJ, Santa Ana CA, et al. Chronic diarrhea of unknown origin. Gastroenterology 1980; 78:264–271.

Tally MJ, Phillips SF, Melton LJ III, et al. A patient questionnaire to identify bowel disease. Ann Intern Med 1989; 111:671–674.

CONSTIPATION

Arvey I. Rogers, M.D.

9

Patients who complain of constipation share a common feature: they are dissatisfied with their bowel movements. Otherwise, the complaint can vary markedly, from patient to patient, in its description. The dissatisfaction may be of recent onset, longstanding, or episodic. The consistency of stools may be described as small, dry, or hard. Some patients may even describe a loose stool as constipation if it is expressed with difficulty. Often these descriptions are associated with a reduction in frequency of defecation, greater than usual effort required to expel stool, or a sensation of incomplete evacuation. Most important to the patient is that a change has occurred in his or her usual bowel habit and consistency of stool. Constipation can occur in any age group; as a rule, women are more apt than men to complain of constipation.

Diarrhea often is thought of as the opposite of constipation, but this is not always the case. In fact, constipation often alternates with diarrhea in the same patient, as in the common irritable bowel syndrome. Seeming even more paradoxic is the "overflow" diarrhea, sometimes with incontinence, that can be a manifestation of a disorder of defecation that actually is constipation complicated by rectal impaction. In this instance, the symptom is diarrhea, but the problem is constipation.

Symptom evaluation by means of a searching history is the oldest and possibly the most reliable tool we have in our diagnostic armamentarium. Only when the patient's complaint has received careful scrutiny can the physician proceed to complete the evaluation in a logical, efficient, cost-effective manner.

On the basis of a sound history, the physician may select from what would otherwise be a bewildering array of available diagnostic techniques (varying in cost, risk, sensitivity, and specificity) those particular tests required to confirm or exclude what is suspected from the history.

The discussion that follows focuses on the evaluation of constipation in the adult. The most meaningful history is obtained from the patient who has the complaint and who is able to communicate its character to the physician. This does not discount the value of observations by perceptive and knowledgeable third parties, such as marital partners, siblings, parents, or caretakers, especially when dealing with a patient who is unwilling or incapable of communicating effectively.

> *"The description of constipation can vary markedly from patient to patient."*

Mechanism of Defecation

Familiarity with the essentials of the anatomic and physiologic aspects of normal defecation is prerequisite to the proper interpretation and evaluation of the symptom of constipation. Such knowledge also provides a rationale for the phrasing and timing of a particular question, as well as interpreting the significance of an answer.

The requirements for normal defecation are summarized in Table 9–1. As described in Chapter 8 "Diarrhea", the small intestine delivers to the colon each day approximately 1 liter of semiliquid residue. By its capacity to absorb water, proportionately equal to that of the small intestine, the colon reduces this residue to about 150 ml, meanwhile transporting the fecal mass distally

> *"Movement of fecal residue through the colon is not a steady passage."*

from the cecum to the sigmoid segment, where it can be held in abeyance until it can be evacuated in a timely and reasonably convenient manner.

Movement of fecal residue along the course of the colon is not a steady passage but rather an intermittent churning, punctuated by relatively infre-

TABLE 9–1. Requirements for Normal Defecation

1. Moist, bulky fecal bolus
2. Stimulus capable of transporting the bolus to the distal colon
3. Normal colon (structurally and functionally)
4. Rectum capable of sensing a normal degree of distention
5. Internal anal sphincter that relaxes reflexly in response to rectal distention
6. Peripheral nervous system capable of responding properly to the distention stimulus and transmitting impulses to the central nervous system
7. Central nervous system capable of responding appropriately to the afferent impulses and preparing the patient psychologically and physically for the act of defecation
8. Conducive physical and psychological environment
9. Ability to maneuver physically into a semisquatting posture, to perform a Valsalva maneuver, and to raise effectively intra-abdominal pressure
10. Desire and ability to evacuate the fecal bolus from the rectum

quent mass propulsive peristalsis. It is important to remember that fecal residue normally is stored in the sigmoid segment, not in the rectum. On digital examination, the rectum should be found nearly empty, except just before evacuation. The finding of a feces-filled rectum at any other time is abnormal.

An urge to stool is triggered by peristaltic propulsion of the fecal mass from the sigmoid colon into the rectum. This pre-evacuatory peristalsis often is initiated by filling of the stomach and is the result of a gastrocolic reflex. Typically, this occurs most forcefully following breakfast or in response to increased physical activity, although some persons may feel an urge to stool following each meal of the day.

> *"Fecal residue normally is stored in the sigmoid colon, not in the rectum."*

Most persons are not quite prepared to defecate immediately on the first impulse generated by the entry of a fecal mass into the rectum. It is at this time that the anal sphincter assumes a role. Contraction of the sphincter allows a limited time for the person to find an acceptable place and posture for the act of defecation. When such a place is found and a squatting posture is assumed, the external anal sphincter can be voluntarily relaxed. Thereupon, the muscular wall of the rectum contracts, and simultaneously the internal anal sphincter relaxes. The fecal mass is thereby extruded. Normally, rectal tension then subsides, yielding a satisfying sensation of having accomplished an essential bowel function.

Most persons are capable of suppressing an urge to stool that is not excessively compelling. When this is done repeatedly, however, there is an eventual dulling of the normal urge to stool despite a full rectum, and this can lead to a common form of constipation.

What to Ask the Constipated Patient

The word *constipation* is in almost everyone's vocabulary, and each patient using the word knows the particular meaning he or she attaches to it. However, this particular meaning has to be elicited and appreciated by the physician. Probably what most people mean is a too infrequent, too difficult passage of a hard stool. But the physician cannot assume, without benefit of further inquiry, that this is always what is meant by the patient who complains, "I'm constipated." It may be that the frequency of bowel movement is unchanged but that the stool has become uncomfortably hard, or that the stool is unchanged but the usual interval between bowel evacuation has become prolonged. Or the patient may simply be lacking an urge to stool, or the urge might be intense but to no avail.

Experience teaches that patients base their complaint of disturbed bowel action by comparison with either their own previous accustomed habit or what they perceive as "normal" in the general population. If the complaint is recent, almost always it is based on a deviation from the patient's own former habit. If the complaint is lifelong, then the patient may be more disturbed by a seeming lack of conformity with general "normalcy" than by difficult bowel movement. The physician has to ask the right questions to learn the basis for the complaint.

When it has been established that a costive change has occurred in the patient's usual stooling pattern, then the single most important question is "Have you lost the urge to stool or do you feel an urge but are unable to comfortably empty the bowel?" If the urge to stool is lacking, then the question is whether this is the result of repeated suppression, or perhaps a disturbance in normal colon transport, or deficiency in fecal bulk. If the urge is intact but evacuation is hampered, then bowel transport and fecal bulk are probably unchanged, and the problem is focused on a disturbance in the anorectal segment. Is there simply no capability of effectively emptying the rectum? Or is the attempt to pass stool hampered by intolerable anal pain? The word *tenesmus,* meaning painful, ineffectual straining at stool, is not in the average patient's vocabulary, and if this is the reason for constipation, it has to be sought by appropriate inquiry. The most common cause is anal fissures.

A frequent reason for a complaint of constipation becomes evident when the patient is asked. "Do you feel comfortable and satisfied after a bowel movement?" Patients whose answer is no often add, "I still feel I have to go." Most often the explanation is persistent hypertonicity in the rectum—that is, failure of the rectal musculature to relax following evacuation. In some cases, this is found due to rectal inflammation. Occasionally the cause is found in a tumor encroaching on the rectal ampulla.

"Repeatedly or habitually suppressing an urge to stool can lead to constipation."

Using the foregoing summary of normal defecation and the vagaries of definition as background, and because a specific complaint should engender a rational list of differential diagnoses based on postulated pathogenesis, varying scenarios are cited in the following sections. Each of these is intended to illustrate one or several explanations of the complaint of constipation. Each is presented in a format somewhat akin to the circumstance of actually obtaining a history—that is, alternating between the data obtained, the analysis of those data, and the elicitation of additional data by the analysis. As each scenario is dissected, a list of differential explanations evolves. Because the list is incomplete, the section is followed by a more detailed tabulation of the causes of constipation (Table 9–2).

TABLE 9–2.   Causes of Constipation

Dietary
   Low fiber intake
   Reduced food intake
   Reduced fluid intake
Medications (see Table 9–3)
Functional
   Physical inactivity
   Weakness
   Immobility
   Depression
   Disorientation
   Non-accommodating toilet facilities
   Physical disability
Secondary Causes
   Metabolic endocrine disorders
   Neuromuscular disorders
   Collagen vascular diseases
   Colonic obstruction

TABLE 9–3.   Medications That May Produce Constipation

Aluminum/calcium antacids
Anticholinergics
Antidepressants
Antihypertensive agents
Antiparkinsonian agents
Antispasmodics
Bismuth-containing preparations
Diuretics (hypokalemia)
Ganglionic blockers
Hematinics (iron)
Narcotic analgesics
Opiates

Confirmation or refutation of suspected causes is usually an easy task, especially when constipation is acute in onset or accompanied by a recognized precipitant, such as the knowing or unknowing use of a constipating agent (Table 9–3). Similarly, the cause may be readily evident by associated symptoms, such as those indicating bowel obstruction. Chronic constipation that has defied previous efforts at diagnosis or has been ineffectively managed may require more sophisticated methods to assess gastrointestinal motility or anorectal function. The concluding section considers some of these methods that can be applied to complete the evaluation of constipation.

Illustrative Case

Data.   A 75-year-old man complained of constipation that had been noted for several months. His normal pattern of a once-daily, soft, formed, spontaneous evacuation following breakfast had diminished to the passage at 3-day intervals of small, hard, difficult-to-evacuate stools. More recently, he noted a sense of rectal fullness and streaks of fresh blood on the toilet paper following difficult evacuation. He also described a sense of incomplete evacuation. There was occasional abdominal cramping preceding an unpredictable urge to defecate.

Analysis.   Obviously, something had happened to affect this man's defecation. The alteration in stool consistency and size suggested diminished fluidity and bulk. The reduced frequency suggested an absence of rectal distention that normally would have provoked a defecatory reflex. The lack of distensive stimulus may have been a consequence of more proximal bowel obstruction that prevented stool from reaching the rectum. Alternatively, the fecal bolus reaching the rectum may have been of insufficient bulk to provoke a defecatory reflex. The difficulty in expelling stool, together with the sense of rectal fullness, the blood streaking the toilet paper, and the feeling of incomplete evacuation suggested the presence of a rectal lesion. The focus initially is on recent events relating to diet, fluid intake, and general health.

Data. It is learned the patient lost 15 pounds in the preceding 4 months, which he attributed to anorexia and reduced food intake. He had been a cigarette smoker for many years. Several years before seeking medical care for constipation he had consulted his internist because of a progressive cough and increasing dyspnea; this led to a diagnosis of chronic obstructive lung disease. In recent months, because of a cough productive of copious and discolored sputum, antibiotics had been prescribed on at least three occasions and for courses of several weeks. The patient also noted that he was more easily fatigued and became dyspneic with minimal effort. He recalled that while taking antibiotics he had been disturbed by anorexia and nausea. This, combined with the burden of pulmonary infection and labored breathing, had led to weight loss.

Analysis. While the foregoing helped to explain some of the change in stooling pattern and consistency, the weight loss and rectal complaints still required further investigation. Was the patient's dyspnea and fatigue of such degree as to impede the act of defecation? Further, how had he reacted to the appearance of blood on the toilet paper?

Data. The patient admitted feeling so weak that he found attempts to defecate increasingly difficult. Seeing blood on the toilet paper aroused anxiety and a fear of cancer. The patient stated that he had preferred to avoid going to stool in order to eliminate this worrisome sight.

Analysis. At this point, it appeared that the patient's complaint of constipation with small, hard stools could be explained in part by reduced intake of food and fluid; that the infrequent urge to defecate and difficulty in expelling stool were the result of dyspnea and weakness consequent to his advanced pulmonary disease; and that this had been compounded by a conscious effort to avoid defecation. The sense of incomplete evacuation could be explained by rectal impaction, and anal bleeding could have resulted from straining at the passage of hard, abrasive stools.

Data. Physical findings confirmed weight loss, generalized weakness, and marked pulmonary impairment. Bowel sounds were active. A segment of feces-filled colon was palpated in the lower left abdomen. Firm feces, which reacted negatively when tested for occult blood, also filled the rectum. Following a cleansing enema, sigmoidoscopy showed no evidence of neoplasm or other mucosal defect. Small internal hemorrhoids were seen in the anal canal. Blood counts and chemical profile were normal.

Diagnosis. Functional constipation, circumstantial, related to associated disease.

The Message. The problem to solve was constipation of recent onset in an elderly man with severe, chronic lung disease. The most likely causes were organic bowel obstruction, the effect of drugs or metabolic disturbance, or a disruption of bowel function consequent to extra-alimentary circumstances. The presence of normal bowel sounds and the absence of abdominal distention, no history of the use of drugs that might suppress bowel movement, and a normal blood chemistry profile and unrevealing proctosigmoidoscopy tended to exclude the first two possibilities. The findings supported the conclusion that the constipation was circumstantial and related to the associated impaired pulmonary function.

Illustrative Case

Data. A 74-year-old woman developed "diarrhea" with fecal soiling during a recent hospitalization for a fractured femur, sustained as a consequence of slipping on icy ground. The patient was immobilized by required traction for 12 days. Parenteral analgesics were required fairly regularly to control pain in the hip, low back (aggravated by chronic arthritis), and right chest (the fifth and sixth ribs also being fractured in the fall). The patient had no bowel movement for the first 10 days of hospitalization and then involuntarily expelled liquid stools for several days. This prompted her attending physician to prescribe a motility suppressant in order to reduce the likelihood of fecal contamination of a "pressure sore" on her left buttock. The patient denied any previous bowel disturbance. She had been given no antibiotics.

Analysis. An explanation for the supposed diarrhea in this patient was not obvious. There was no indication of intestinal infection. Liquid stool seeping from the anus contained no white blood cells or occult blood. Physical examination was hampered by the patient's immobility, but no abnormalities were encountered except for some loss of skin turgor and a dry mouth. A laboratory report of highly concentrated urine and elevated blood urea nitrogen pointed to the possibility of dehydration resulting from reduced fluid intake and presumed diarrhea. Intravenous fluids were recommended. Motility suppressants continued to be given "as needed to control the diarrhea."

Data. The problem of "loose stools" and fecal soiling of the bed sheets continued despite the use of motility suppressants. Abdominal cramping prompted a request for a scout film of the abdomen. This revealed a moderate amount of gas distributed throughout an otherwise normal proximal colon; more surprising was the appearance of a feces-filled left colon.

Analysis. In sifting through the data thus far obtained it was found, with dismay, that a rectal examination had been omitted. The explanation was that the patient's immobility and weakened condition had precluded this. Moreover, the absence of blood in the stools mitigated concern for a rectal lesion.

Data. The omission was corrected. The examiner's gloved finger encountered a large, hard, fecal mass filling the rectal ampulla. The patient remarked that rectal manipulation reproduced a pressure sensation she had felt several times during her hospitalization.

Diagnosis. Paradoxic diarrhea due to fecal impaction of the rectum.

The Message. In retrospect, the patient was "set up" for the occurrence of fecal impaction. She was immobilized, dehydrated, and receiving constipating analgesics. An early clue, unfortunately overlooked, was the lack of bowel movements during the first week or so of her hospitalization. That she did not complain of uncomfortable rectal pressure may be explained by the regular administration of analgesic medication, which dulled her sensation. Had a rectal examination been performed earlier, the diagnosis could have been established. Failure to do so not only delayed diagnosis but also aggravated the condition by permitting the continued use of motility suppressants. Graver consequences might have ensued had the problem remained unsolved. It is well to remember that one of the most common causes of apparent diarrhea in an elderly, immobilized patient is actually constipation leading to fecal impaction.

Illustrative Case

Data. A 30-year-old woman, stated "I am constipated all the time. I never go to the bathroom unless I take a laxative, which I have to do at least once a week to relieve my bloating. And I never get an urge anymore."

She had seen many physicians about this problem, which began during puberty or late teens and became worse when the patient was a full-time law student. Endoscopic and radiographic examinations had been reported as "normal." The use of traditional bulk laxatives, "stool softeners," and increased dietary fiber were of no avail. She varied her weekly laxative regimen to avoid "dependency."

Analysis. The presentation was that of a young woman whose chronic constipation was of obscure cause. It was deemed important to review films of her most recent barium enema examination, looking for any colonic dilatation that might suggest organic or functional obstruction. Her generally healthy appearance made one wonder about her diet, fluid intake, and stool habits over the years. Because appearances can be deceiving, a search should be made for clues of masked depression or anxiety. The purposeful or inadvertent use of constipating medications (see Table 9–3) also should be considered. In a young woman, as in this case, inquiry directed at possible pelvic trauma, as from a previous difficult delivery or surgery, would additionally be merited.

Data. It is learned that the patient is a member of a prominent law firm and is "busy constantly." Beginning in her late teens and continuing through her time at law school, the patient frequently ignored the urge to stool because "it always came at the wrong time and in the wrong place." A pattern that had allowed the bowel to move daily or every other day gave way to a delayed frequency of every 3 to 5 days until the past few years when "weeks go by without an urge." She has had no previous pelvic surgery and is nulliparous. She has been married for 4 years to a fellow attorney. The couple uses no contraceptive device. She admits to feeling depressed sometimes because she has not yet conceived. Still, she has been preoccupied by the demands of her profession, protesting that "I never have enough time to get my work done."

The patient has taken no medication on a regular basis, although at one time she had been advised that her thyroid gland was "underactive" and that this might have contributed to earlier weight gain. She admitted to eating irregularly and "on the run." The bulk of her caloric intake was consumed in the evenings when she and her husband ate "late dinners" while watching television. She tended to avoid fiber-containing foods because they "make me gassy." She had no time for exercise and devoted her weekends to "just relaxing."

Analysis. It was clear that the patient's poor eating habits could predispose to insufficient bulk. She denied herself the benefit of proper exercise. Her frantic work schedule doubtless contributed to stress and may have inclined her to depression. What about the patient's systems review and family history?

Data. The patient admitted occasional difficulty in initiating urination. Her hands were "always cold," and she sometimes became "light-headed" for no apparent reason. She had regular menses, although plagued by severe dysmenorrhea since puberty. She denied changes in skin texture or undue intolerance of cold temperatures. She was aware of no family history of alimentary or neuromuscular disorders.

Physical examination was unrevealing. Notable was an undistended abdomen with normal bowel sounds. Anorectal examination disclosed a few, small, hemorrhoidal tags and a rectum containing soft feces. Blood counts, complete chemistry profile, and measures of thyroid function were unremarkable. Barium enema showed an anatomically intact colon.

Analysis.   These data essentially excluded from consideration anal stenosis, Hirschsprung's disease (long- and short-segment types), and other causes of bowel obstruction (hernia, tumor, stricture, volvulus), metabolic and endocrine disorders (hypothyroidism, diabetes, hypercalcemia, panhypopituitarism), neuropathy, muscular disorders, collagen-vascular disease, and iatrogenic causes of constipation.

Complaints of cold hands, lightheadedness, and difficulty urinating have been related to a syndrome of chronic constipation in young women that has been described as "idiopathic slow-transit constipation." The finding or a rectum filled with stool of sufficient bulk to ordinarily provoke an urge to defecation suggested dysfunction of the anorectal segment.

Data.   The patient was convinced of the need for investigation of bowel transit by means of radiopaque markers ingested after the colon and rectum had been properly emptied by thorough cleansing. In this test, 50 percent of the markers were retained in the rectum after 5 days (normally less than 20 percent are retained); during the study period the patient denied urge to stool or actual defecation.

Anorectal manometry was performed after the rectum had been completely decompressed. Distention of the rectum produced no urge to defecate even when the volume introduced exceeded that normally required (less than 30 ml). The patient was unable to evacuate a balloon filled with 150 ml of a weak barium suspension. The expected relaxation of the internal anal sphincter in response to rectal distention (the rectoanal inhibitory reflex) was observed. Finally, electromyography of the pelvic floor revealed a paradoxic increase in tension of the puborectalis muscle when the patient attempted to defecate.

Analysis.   Of the above studies, it would have sufficed to determine by the position of bowel transit markers that there was no diffuse disorder of colonic motility. The demonstration by anorectal manometry of an intact rectoanal inhibitory reflex excluded Hirschsprung's disease and obviated any need to show the characteristic absence of ganglion cells and increased tissue levels of acetylcholinesterase by full-thickness biopsy of the rectal wall.

Diagnosis.   Idiopathic chronic constipation, with abnormal rectal motility and possible spasm of the puborectalis muscle.

The Message.   Many possible causes require consideration and exclusion before assigning a label of "idiopathic chronic constipation." A thorough history, including that of past medical events, previous medication, personal habits, family background, and complete systems review, combined with physical examination and a few selected laboratory tests, should enable the clinician to arrive at a correct diagnosis.

Studies of gastrointestinal motility have suggested there are at least four patterns of altered function (described below along with appropriate tests) that can be identified in patients with chronic constipation of obscure origin. Unfortunately, characterization of these disorders does not always ensure success in their medical management.

"Many possibilities must be considered before assigning the label 'idiopathic chronic' to constipation."

Remarks on the Pathophysiology of Constipation as Illustrated in the Foregoing Scenarios

Having completed the history and physical examination, the clinician should be able to postulate a reasonable explanation for the patient's complaint of constipation. Answers to the following questions should be forthcoming: Which requirements for effective defecation have or have not been met? What primary or secondary causes might there be for failure to meet these requirements?

In Case 1, the problem was focused on the adequacy of the fecal bolus, the stimulus to defecation, the ability to physically maneuver, and the desire to evacuate the rectum. The patient's food and fluid intake had diminished (reducing the fecal bolus); his physical activity was curtailed (inhibiting the stimulus); his strength was depleted (impairing the effort required for defecation); and he suppressed an urge to stool to lessen the anxiety engendered by the appearance of blood on the toilet paper.

In Case 2, constipation presented as paradoxic diarrhea. Out of misguided concern for the patient's debility, exploration of the rectum was omitted from the initial physical examination. Failure to appreciate that what appears to be diarrhea may be a manifestation of rectal fecal impaction misdirected attention to the loose stools. This, in turn, led to well-meant but ill-advised efforts to suppress "diarrhea." These only aggravated the underlying constipation that was abetted by immobilization, physical incapacity, reduced food and fluid intake, motility-inhibiting medications, and drug-dulled sensory input. In this case, of the 10 requirements for normal stooling listed in Table 9–1, eight were not met.

In Case 3, chronic constipation was the bane of a busy young female attorney. There were no obviously contributing factors other than neglected bowel habit and reduced bulk and fluid intake. Circumstantial and physical evaluations were unrevealing. Further objective assessment, including anorectal manometry, disclosed abnormality in requirements 4 and 10 in Table 9–1. It is not certain whether these defects are cause or consequence, but they appear to be implicated in the patient's complaint.

Before embarking on more involved tests, it is useful to construct a rational list of probable or possible causes for constipation by consideration of the following:

1. Is the patient in vigorous youth or midlife, or is the patient elderly and debilitated?
2. Is the constipation recent or longstanding?
3. What are the circumstances in which constipation has occurred?
4. Which requirements for effective defecation (see Table 9–1) are lacking?
5. Has bleeding been noted with bowel movements?
6. Is bowel evacuation painful?
7. What medications or associated disorders or diseases may have contributed to impaired defecation?
8. What special diagnostic tests are required to confirm the clinical impression derived from analysis of deficient requirements for effective defecation?

Diagnostic Options

Assuming a thorough history and physical examination have been recorded and that urinalysis, hemogram, and blood chemistry profile have been obtained, how should further evaluation proceed?

- Proctosigmoidoscopy should be considered part of the routine physical examination for any patient complaining of constipation. Regardless of clinical impressions, it is essential to determine the presence or absence of a mucosal lesion in the distal colon or anorectum. This procedure also allows for biopsy.

> *"Proctosigmoidoscopy should be considered part of the examination of any patient complaining of constipation."*

- If metabolic, endocrine, or collagen-vascular disorders are suspected, hormone assays or serologic (antibody) tests should be performed.
- If colonic obstruction, either structural or functional, is suspected, a scout film of the abdomen should be performed.

- Barium enema examination is not always necessary but should be done if obstruction is suspected and proctosigmoidoscopy has disclosed no lesion in the distal segment. Colonoscopy is unnecessary in the usual case of constipation; it should be reserved for those instances in which a proximal lesion is otherwise suspected. Some clinicians prefer it over barium enema.
- A colon transit study can be helpful when there is no obvious explanation for constipation. This study requires a thoroughly cleansed colon, together with a high-residue diet and adequate fluid intake during the

---

*"**B**owel transit may be assessed through the use of ingested radiopaque markers."*

---

procedure. Radiopaque markers to be ingested can be homemade or commercially obtained. The progress of markers through the alimentary canal is determined by single or serial plain films of the abdomen, thus showing how many markers remain and where they are distributed. Normally, more than 80 percent of markers should have been evacuated after 5 to 7 days. Diffuse distribution in the colon of abnormally retained markers suggests altered neuromuscular function, which may be limited to the colon or may affect the entire gastrointestinal tract. An excess of markers clustered in the distal colon is evidence of impaired perception of the fecal mass, often in a setting of emotional disturbance. Markers retained in the lowermost segment point to anorectal outlet obstruction.
- Anorectal manometry, utilizing a triple-balloon or water-perfused system, enables assessment of threshold for rectal sensing of a fecal bolus and also whether the rectoanal inhibitory reflex is intact. Hirschsprung's disease is suspected when the internal anal sphincter fails to relax in response to rectal distention. The ability to spontaneously evacuate a balloon distended with up to 150 ml of a semisolid substance tests rectal and anal function. Some radiology departments perform defecography, a cinefluoroscopic and radiographic recording of rectal and anal function, using a semisolid radiopaque bolus. Electromyography of the anorectal and pelvic musculature can be obtained, but the method is not widely available and results may be difficult to interpret.
- If a diffuse gastrointestinal neuromuscular disorder is suspected, esophageal manometry and gastric emptying tests may be in order.
- Varying rectosigmoid response to meals and edrophonium may be helpful in differentiating certain motility disorders, as suggested in a recent report by Reynolds and colleagues (Table 9–4).

TABLE 9-4. Rectosigmoid Responses in Patients with Chronic Constipation and Motility Abnormalities

Pattern	Rectosigmoid Response	
	To Meal	To Tensilon
Anal sphincter dysfunction	Normal	Normal
Colonic inertia*	Reduced	Normal
Diffuse gastrointestinal motor disorder	Reduced	Reduced
Irritable bowel syndrome*	Increased	Increased

Modified from Reynolds JC, Ouyang A, Lee CA, et al. Chronic severe constipation: Prospective motility studies in 25 consecutive patients. Gastroenterology 1987; 92:414-420.
*Anorectal manometry is normal.

- Useful information can be obtained by simply eliminating or modifying circumstances or conditions that can affect requirements for effective defecation (see Table 9-1).

To Sum Up

Like almost all symptoms, constipation lends itself to thorough analysis through history and physical examination. Obtaining data and interpreting it properly should enable the physician to determine which of the requirements for effective defecation are impaired and to be able, in turn, to relate these correctly to the clinical setting. Only then can a reasonable list of causes be postulated as a basis for rational selection of the few diagnostic tests required to confirm the clinical impression.

Suggested Reading

Brocklehurst JC. Colonic disease in the elderly. Clin Gastroenterol 1985; 14:725-747.

Devroede G, Poisson J, Schang J-C. Obstipation: What is the appropriate therapeutic approach? In: Barkin JS, Rogers AI, eds. Difficult decisions in digestive diseases. Chicago: Year Book, 1989:458-484.

Preston DM, Lennard-Jones JE. Severe chronic constipation of young women: "Idiopathic slow transit constipation." Gut 1986; 27:41-48.

Preston DM, Lennard-Jones JE, Thomas BM. The balloon proctogram. Br J Surg 1984; 71:29-32.

Read NW. Constipation. In: Bayless TM, ed. Current therapy in gastroenterology and liver disease. 3rd ed. Philadelphia: BC Decker, 1990:324-327.

Read NW, Timms JM. Defecation and the pathophysiology of constipation. Clin Gastroenterol 1986; 15:937-965.

Read NW, Timms JM, Barfield LJ, et al. Impairment of defecation in young women with severe constipation. Gastroenterology 1986; 90:53-60.

Reynolds JC, Ouyang A, Lee CA, et al. Chronic severe constipation: Prospective motility studies in 25 consecutive patients. Gastroenterology 1987; 92:414-420.

Wald A. Colonic transit and anorectal manometry in chronic idiopathic constipation. Arch Intern Med 1986; 146:1713–1716.

Wald A. Colorectal function and constipation in the elderly. Pract Gastroenterol 1989; 13:36, 41, 46–47.

Whitehead WE, Schuster MM. Manometric and electromyographic techniques for assessment of the anorectal mechanism for continence and defecation. In: Hoelzl R, Whitehead WE, eds. Psychophysiology of the gastrointestinal tract: Experimental and clinical applications. New York: Plenum, 1983:321–329.

JAUNDICE

Henry J. Tumen, M.D.

10

The jaundiced patient brings to the physician a diagnostic problem that often is difficult to resolve but is always interesting and challenging. Assembling the various items of diagnostic information needed to define the cause of jaundice may be compared with putting together a complicated jigsaw puzzle. There is the same urge to put each piece in place, particularly to fill in the last blank space, to see all dimensions of the clinical problem, and to learn how it all fits together. But, just as a jigsaw puzzle cannot be solved by dropping the pieces at random on the board, so determining the cause of a patient's jaundice requires careful evaluation and integration of every bit of information as it is acquired.

There also must be a foundation on which to assemble that information. This foundation is best established by a detailed review of the patient's medical history, past and present, along with a competent physical examination, supplemented by a few readily obtained, basic laboratory examinations. There is much evidence, however, that a clinical diagnosis of the cause of jaundice, arrived at without recourse to any laboratory tests and based solely on analysis of the history and physical examination, probably will be confirmed by subsequent, more elaborate procedures.[1,2] It is recommended, therefore, that involved and invasive studies be undertaken only after a logical, tentative clinical diagnosis of the cause of jaundice has been postulated. If done then, such studies will be more helpful in resolving the diagnosis, with a saving of time and expense. Also, the risks that some invasive procedures entail will be avoided.

Jaundice, of itself, should not create a sense of diagnostic urgency or call for hasty diagnostic exertions. A well-planned, discriminating approach to determining the origin of jaundice in a given patient is more likely to lead to resolution of the patient's problem than is a pell-mell, "all-the-tests-in-the-book" assault.

Mechanisms of Jaundice

Jaundice is the outward manifestation of many different disorders that lead to an increase in serum bilirubin levels sufficient to give a distinctive yellow tint to the skin, sclerae, almost all body tissues, and, when bilirubin is principally in a conjugated or soluble form, the urine. Bilirubin is the normal end product of catabolism of heme that is, for the most part, released from erythrocytes as they disintegrate at the end of their normal life span of 120 days. A lesser amount derives from the breakdown of hemoproteins in liver and muscle.

A vital and important intermediary step in the catabolism of heme is its conversion to biliverdin in phagocytic cells of the liver, spleen, and bone marrow (Fig. 10–1). Within the same cells the biliverdin is rapidly changed to bilirubin by further enzymatic action. Bilirubin, at first bound to albumin, is taken up by the hepatocytes (the parenchymal cells of the liver) and under-

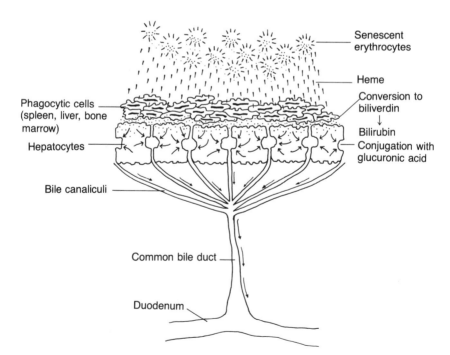

FIGURE 10–1. Diagrammatic depiction of the origin, metabolism, transport, and excretion of bilirubin.

goes a process of conjugation whereby bilirubin is linked, for the most part, to glucuronic acid through the action of intracellular enzymes. Conjugation makes bilirubin water-soluble and permits its passage through cell walls into intercellular biliary ductules and thence through progressively larger excretory passages to the common bile duct and finally to the intestine. The process of progressive catabolic changes of heme to biliverdin and then to bilirubin results in the daily production of about 4 mg per kilogram of bilirubin, with fairly constant levels of bilirubin in the serum of about 1 mg per deciliter. Of the serum bilirubin, about 0.1 mg per deciliter is normally in the conjugated ("direct reacting") form; the remainder is unconjugated ("indirect reacting").

It can be seen from this brief description of the formation and excretion of bilirubin that interference with any of the integrated sequential steps may lead to hyperbilirubinemia and to jaundice. One possibility is disintegration of erythrocytes at an abnormally rapid rate, as occurs in hemolytic anemia. This results in liberation of large amounts of heme (the parent substance) and, from this, the production of bilirubin in quantities exceeding the conjugated and excretory capacities of normal hepatocytes. In contrast, disease or dysfunction of the liver cells may reduce their ability to conjugate and excrete bilirubin, even in the quantity normally formed. Either of these circumstances will result in hyperbilirubinemia. Another possibility is that bilirubin may be produced, conjugated, and excreted from the liver in normal quantities and begin its passage through the biliary duct system, only to have bile flow impeded by an obstructive lesion, such as a stone, tumor, or stricture. Any impediment in bile flow causes intraductal pressure to rise and leads to resorption of conjugated bilirubin into lymph and blood channels. Again, the net result is hyperbilirubinemia and jaundice.

This definition and interpretation of the mechanisms that can cause hyperbilirubinemia led McNee, in 1923, to suggest that jaundice may be classified according to whether its origin was *hemolytic, hepatocellular,* or *obstructive.*[3] This classification rapidly gained acceptance and popular use; its terminology was simple and easy to define. Moreover, it conformed to the then current understanding of liver physiology and the pathogenesis of jaundice, and it seemed to be of value in planning therapeutic strategy. However, growing knowledge has revealed inadequacies in McNee's classification. One reason is that clinical jaundice often is the consequence of multiple factors. Elements of hemolysis, liver cell injury, and biliary obstruction can coexist, and each can contribute to the manifestation of jaundice. A major defect in the older classification is that it does not fully take into account the process now recognized as "cholestasis," a condition in which bile flow ceases or stops.[4]

Another frequently used classification divides jaundice into *prehepatic, hepatic,* and *posthepatic* types. This arrangement has the advantage of focusing consideration of possible etiologic factors on the basic anatomic locations where these factors would be operative.

Understanding of the pathogenesis of cholestasis has expanded rapidly in recent years. Bile flow may be impeded by obstruction involving primarily the major bile ducts (extrahepatic cholestasis), a common and well-recognized clinical problem. It is now known that cholestasis also may be caused by dysfunction in the excretory membranes of the liver cells themselves (intra-hepatic cholestasis). This cellular dysfunction is highly selective in that it does not diminish the capacity of hepatocytes to conjugate bilirubin, but it does decrease their ability to excrete bilirubin after its conjugation.

The pathogenesis of selective dysfunction of the hepatocytes is a subject of ongoing investigation of hepatocyte physiology. Attention has focused on al-tered permeability of the membranes that form the walls of the hepatocytes, particularly those from which arise the tiny bile canaliculi that constitute the very beginning of the biliary excretory system. The permeability of these membranes may be greatly influenced by changes in the bile acids them-selves, resulting from the action of various toxic substances, drugs, and hor-mones. Much still remains to be learned, however, about the mechanisms of cholestasis.

For the clinician faced with the problem of determining the cause of jaundice in a given case, it is important to know that liver cell injury and dysfunction, with altered cell wall permeability, can result in jaundice that assumes a "cholestatic" character. What constitutes primarily a hepatocellular disturbance can produce jaundice similar in many respects to the obstructive jaundice caused by gross blockage of the biliary tract. The differentiation, therefore, between cholestatic jaundice due to hepatocellular dysfunction and that caused by extrahepatic biliary obstruction is a major diagnostic problem.

Diagnostic Approach to Jaundice

Medical History

Eliciting a thorough medical history is the essential first step in the diagnostic approach to the patient who appears to be jaundiced. Experience has shown that information derived from the patient is the single most helpful guide to establishing the cause of jaundice.

The first and most obvious point: Is the patient a man or a woman? Gender imposes differing, if not distinctive, liability to various forms of jaundice. If the patient is a man, the focus should be on tumors and liver damage, particularly as related to alcohol abuse; if the patient is a woman, cholelithiasis should be considered. Is the patient young or old? Age alone points to likely and unlikely categories of jaundice. In younger persons, the possibility of hepatitis in one of its forms comes to mind; in older persons, tumor and gallstone disease should be considered the paramount possibilities. Does the patient appear acutely ill, chronically ill, or simply yellow and not ill at all?

Three aspects of the patient's history require careful notation:

1. The duration and course of jaundice since its onset.

2. Symptoms or signs coincident with jaundice.
3. Inquiry of previous factors or circumstances possibly contributory to jaundice.

The Course of Jaundice.   Has jaundice been longstanding (weeks, months, or years) or only recently noted (days or hours)? Was the apparent onset abrupt (skin clear one day, then lemon-yellow the next)? Or was the onset of jaundice uncertain and barely perceptible? In the latter case, was the urine discolored before the color change in the skin was noted? It is a curious fact that often the patient will have been at first unaware of icterus and will have been informed of his or her yellow cast only by a family member or friend. Is the yellowness of the skin and eyes and the discoloration of the urine deepening or diminishing? Here again, the observation of a companion may be more reliable than that of the patient. Has jaundice been persistent or intermittent? If intermittent, has the jaundice completely disappeared or merely waned? How long have been the intervals between episodes of jaundice?

> **"S**trangely, icterus that is obvious to someone else may be inapparent to the patient."

Symptoms or Signs Coincident with Jaundice.   Of immediate concern is concomitant pain that typically, but not always, marks biliary obstruction. The one situation that may call for urgency is the need to relieve an obstructive lesion causing extrahepatic cholestasis, the two most frequent conditions being calculous biliary tract disease and carcinoma at or near the head of the pancreas.

Questions should be asked about the occurrence in the past of attacks of pain suggestive of gallstones (see Chapter 2, "Abdominal Pain"). Typically, these attacks are described by the patient as irregularly occurring episodes of severe pain in the epigastrium and right upper abdomen, possibly associated with fever and darkening of the urine. Inquiry should be made about previous diagnostic studies that may have been carried out following an earlier attack. Did oral cholecystography disclose a nonfunctioning gallbladder, or did ultrasonography show the presence of gallstones? If an earlier attack led to surgical intervention, one should obtain a complete operative report. Were stones actually found? Where? Was the common bile duct explored? Although the patient may not be able to supply all of these answers, he or she can often help. For example, the patient will know if a drain or catheter was left protruding from the abdomen after operation. If the patient does not know the difference between a drain and a catheter, ask how long the device was left in place. If it was removed after only a few days, it probably was a drain; if it was not withdrawn until 2 or 3 weeks had passed, it most likely was a T-tube catheter. If a catheter was in place, was it clamped to stop external drainage before it was removed? Did clamping result in pain or recurrence of jaundice? Was a solution injected and a radiograph taken before the catheter was withdrawn?

When patients complain of recurrent pain or jaundice following cholecystectomy and exploration of the common bile duct, there is always a question whether the symptoms are caused by residual or recurrent biliary stones, or are due to stricture of the common bile duct. Stricture, the less likely cause, usually is manifest within months or little more than a year after operation, whereas a problem with residual or recurrent stones may become evident as early as a few weeks or as late as many years. The longer the interval between biliary tract surgery and the onset of pain with jaundice, the greater the likelihood that the cause is stone rather than stricture. Also, once symptoms due to stricture begin, they are usually more persistent than symptoms caused by stone, which tend to be intermittent with typically lengthy symptom-free intervals. "Painless jaundice" was thought in the past to characterize carcinoma of the pancreas, but this is now known to be the case in only a small minority of patients. Jaundice may precede pain when an early carcinoma impinges on the common bile duct but remains confined to the head of the pancreas. When carcinoma arises in the body or tail of the pancreas, jaundice is a relatively late symptom, becoming evident only weeks or months following the onset of pain, weight loss, and debility. Whether early or late, jaundice associated with pancreatic carcinoma almost invariably persists and steadily increases.

Acute pain of a typically hepatobiliary distribution is a frequent concomitant of cholestatic jaundice in cases of "ascending cholangitis" due to any cause. In these instances, jaundice and pain are almost concurrent.

> *"Truly painless jaundice suggests hemolysis, intrahepatic cholestasis, or certain unusual neoplasms."*

Truly painless jaundice occurs in hemolysis, in most cases of intrahepatic cholestasis (including that of primary biliary cirrhosis), in some cases of hepatitis, and in the earlier phases of cholangiocarcinoma and carcinoma arising in the duodenal ampulla of Vater. Jaundice associated with cholangiocarcinoma, once evident, tends to persist; jaundice occurring with ampullary tumors may be intermittent. Jaundice due to drugs whose side effect is "pure" cholestasis is almost always painless. Most patients with acute viral hepatitis are preoccupied with the malaise of their illness, and many complain of soreness in the right hypochondrium; their icterus concerns them less. However, there is a type of hepatitis that is predominantly cholestatic, and for these patients jaundice, without pain, is the principal symptom.

Fever typically accompanies the jaundice of hepatitis and cholangitis. In hepatitis the fever is usually of low or moderate degree. In suppurative cholangitis, fever can reach high, spiking peaks. Fever of varying degree also is typical of jaundice associated with hemolysis when pyrogenic substances are released along with heme from disintegrating red blood cells.

Itching is a common concomitant of cholestatic jaundice, especially that associated with carcinoma of the pancreas and cholestatic hepatitis. In such cases, annoying itching may precede the patient's awareness of icterus. Similarly, itching often precedes visible jaundice and may remain the preponderant symptom in patients with primary biliary cirrhosis. Itching can affect all skin surfaces but often is felt more intensely in the palms of the hands and the soles of the feet. Most patients find the pruritus of cholestasis more troublesome at night, probably because they are not otherwise distracted and possibly because of the effect of heat from bed coverings. In many cases, the physician is obliged to elicit specifically the symptom of itching; it is often not volunteered by the patient.

Anorexia, nausea, and vomiting, while fairly common in the jaundiced patient, are not induced by hyperbilirubinemia alone and, if present, are not commensurate with the level of serum bilirubin. They are symptoms of underlying disease, of which jaundice may be only another manifestation (see Chapter 5, "Nausea and Vomiting"; Chapter 13, "Anorexia"; and Chapter 14, "Eating Disorders").

Weight loss associated with jaundice, especially when both symptoms are protracted, usually points to neoplasia. This is particularly true of carcinoma of the pancreas (see Chapter 2, "Abdominal Pain"; and Chapter 7, "Weight Loss"). Anorexia accompanying the jaundice of acute hepatitis often leads to a short-term drop in weight that, in most cases, is promptly regained on recovery.

Changes in the color of urine and feces are perhaps more accurately considered as signs rather than symptoms, but significant information pertaining to these changes can be elicited from the patient. A change in the color of urine from its normal straw-yellow to orange or amber is noticed more often by the patient than is a change in the color of feces from brown to greasy-gray. Frank steatorrhea as a result of cholestasis is relatively infrequent. When inquiring about the urine, it is best to avoid leading questions. One should ask "Have you noticed any unusual color in your urine?" rather than "Has your urine been dark?" It can be helpful to offer comparisons by asking "Is your urine the color of strong tea or as dark as a cola drink?" If the patient claims that the urine looked dark, ask at what time of day this was observed. One can be misled by a report of normally darker, concentrated urine passed after arising from a night's sleep. Hyperbilirubinuria of cholestasis is apparent throughout the day and deeply tints the toilet-bowl water when only a small volume of urine has been passed. It also is worth glancing at the patient's underpants. Even a few drops of bilirubin-tainted urine can produce telltale spots. Better yet, obtain a specimen of the patient's urine, and inspect it yourself. Interestingly, when the patient's attention is called to darkening of urine, it will be found that this observation preceded an awareness of icterus; conversely, a waning icterus often is preceded by lightening of the color of urine.

Significant Past Medical History.   Mention has been made of the need to inquire carefully about circumstances pertaining to previous experience with calculous biliary tract disease. When there has been previous surgical intervention, it is best to solicit actual copies of the surgeon's and pathologist's reports. Meanwhile, as noted earlier, a good deal of helpful information can be obtained by questioning the patient.

"Amber urine, as a sign of cholestasis, often is noticed before icterus is apparent."

Inquiry should be made about possible exposure to infectious diseases and about exotic travel. The list of infectious diseases that may be accompanied by jaundice is well known, and many of these are infections to which travelers to foreign countries are particularly susceptible. It is also important to elicit a history of blood transfusion or injection of blood products, no matter how remote in time. Our current culture is such that one is obliged to inquire frankly about the illicit use of needles and the patient's sexual proclivity.

A past history of symptoms suggesting chronic inflammatory bowel disease, particularly idiopathic ulcerative colitis, points to the possibility of jaundice that is due to supervening cholangitis, typically of the secondary, sclerosing type.[5] In most cases, evidence of ulcerative colitis precedes that of sclerosing cholangitis. A previous colectomy does not preclude this complication. The jaundice of sclerosing cholangitis may not appear until after the inflamed colon has been resected. The symptoms of primary sclerosing cholangitis, including recurrent bouts of jaundice, pain, and fever, are often similar to those of calculous biliary tract disease.[6]

Clues may be obtained from the family history. In a jaundiced patient suspected of infectious disease, one would be concerned with the occurrence of similar symptoms in another family member, particularly a sexual partner.

A familial disorder associated with jaundice that is a frequent cause of unwarranted concern is Gilbert's syndrome. This is a clinically innocent form of low-grade hyperbilirubinemia that may reach levels of frank jaundice coincident with periods of excessive fatigue or minor systemic infections. Often Gilbert's syndrome is revealed incidentally when slight hyperbilirubinemia is reported in a comprehensive panel of blood chemistry tests obtained for unrelated reasons. The defect is an inability of hepatocytes to conjugate bilirubin; hence the elevation in total serum bilirubin (usually less than 3 mg per deciliter) is almost entirely in the unconjugated component. Liver function is otherwise unimpaired, and the condition is compatible with a normally healthy life span. To recognize Gilbert's syndrome, alerted by a family history, is to allay undue anxiety and avoid unnecessary investigation and futile therapeutic ventures.

In assessing the jaundiced patient, it is of utmost importance to compile a complete record of exposure to potentially hepatotoxic drugs. First and foremost is the need to determine the patient's past and recent use of alcohol. Jaundice is a late symptom of most forms of chronic, alcohol-induced liver injury, such as cirrhosis; however, jaundice may be among the initial, acute symptoms of alcholic hepatitis, a devastating affliction typically seen in a setting of malnutrition and triggered by an alcoholic debauch. The extent to which previous consumption of alcohol may contribute to liability to jaundice from other causes is uncertain.

The list of medications that may cause jaundice as a side effect or adverse reaction is almost endless. Some drugs predictably produce a dose-related hyperbilirubinemia. More often, jaundice occurs sporadically in only a minority of users, presumably because of individual susceptibility. Some drugs produce only intrahepatic cholestasis; some can induce the equivalent of diffuse hepatitis; some drugs do both. Usually, the offending drug will have been taken shortly before the appearance of jaundice, but the interval between the use of a drug and its adverse effect is not always predictable.

One should be mindful that certain drugs can color urine bright yellow or orange and yet be unassociated with hyperbilirubinemia. Typical examples are the azo dyes, notably pyridium, and also B-complex vitamins when taken in excessive doses. Quinacrine (Atabrine) is an intensely yellow substance that when taken for long periods, as in prophylaxis for malaria, gives the skin and eyeballs a yellow cast.

Needless to say, because a drug has been taken and jaundice ensues does not establish a cause-and-effect relation. However, because chemically induced jaundice is common and often unpredictable, a thorough accounting of all medications and exposure to potentially noxious substances is essential to the medical history.

Inquiry also should be directed to recent digestion of shellfish, which may have been contaminated with hepatitis virus; to contact with aquaria in which turtles may have shed hepatitis virus; to exposure to wild or pet animals that may have been ill; and to recent injections with possibly contaminated needles.

Physical Examination

Jaundice may be immediately and unquestionably visible but, just as faint icterus may have escaped notice by the patient, it may be difficult for the physician to discern. It is important to view the patient in a proper light. A well-illuminated examining room is usually satisfactory, but examination by natural daylight is by far the best. Individual characteristics of the patient can pose a problem. The skin of dark-complexioned persons does not readily betray icterus. The level of hyperbilirubinemia detectable by visual inspection in the average person of fair complexion is depicted in Figure 10–2.

> *"Look at the periphery of the orbit for the most intense scleral icterus."*

When hyperbilirubinemia is relatively slight, it is essential to know where to look for jaundice. The skin of the face and hands, normally pigmented by exposure to sunlight, often is misleading; the skin of the abdomen is the place to look. The normally white sclerae of the eyes readily reflect the yellow tinge of bilirubin, but the redness of conjunctivitis or the brown tint of melanin can make this less easily discernible. Yellow tinting of the sclerae by bilirubin is much more pronounced in the periphery of the eyeballs than adjacent to the iris. This contrasts with staining by photosensitizing drugs, such as quinacrine (Atabrine), which is more evident in portions of the sclerae not covered by the eyelids and hence exposed to sunlight. Because of this, discoloration by photosensitizing agents can be readily distinguished from actual jaundice. This can be important in patients with a history of prophylactic use of quinacrine and exposure to endemic, icterogenic disease. As mentioned previously, if yellowness of the skin is unmistakable, and yet the sclerae are clearly white, the diagnosis is carotenemia, not jaundice. One can look at the oral mucosa under the tongue, but this is seldom helpful if icterus is uncertain elsewhere.

The degree of jaundice sometimes is a clue to its origin. The most intense icterus is more likely to occur with cholestasis, particularly of the intrahepatic type, rather than with hepatocellular disease. There is a limit to jaundice. Rarely, if ever, does hyperbilirubinemia exceed 40 mg per deciliter. Therefore, even though obstruction becomes complete, the degree of jaundice and the level of serum bilirubin does not change once a peak has been reached.

Clinicians of a bygone era were fond of ascribing diagnostic significance to particular hues of jaundice, and these variants are still worth noting. The brightest yellow is seen in the glow of a patient with acute intrahepatic cholestasis. A sallow, greenish-yellow typifies the complexion of a patient with

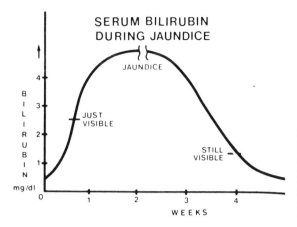

FIGURE 10-2. Correlation of visible jaundice with serum bilirubin concentrations. (Reprinted with permission from Schaffner F. Jaundice. In: Berk JE, Haubrich WS, Kalsner H, Roth JLA, Schaffner F, eds. Bockus Gastroenterology. 4th ed. Philadelphia: WB Saunders, 1985: 168.

more longstanding jaundice, such as that occurring in advanced cirrhosis. A distinctly chartreuse tinge, particularly when observed in an older patient who itches and whose abdominal examination discloses a palpable gallbladder, clearly points to an obstructing lesion in or about the head of the pancreas. The conventional, perhaps oversimplified, explanation for the green tint is oxidation of bilirubin to its precursor biliverdin. This reversion can occur in stagnant bile that has been invaded by bacteria. Absorption of green-colored biliverdin is thought to give the skin and other tissues the characteristically variant hue.

Much has been made, too, of purportedly distinctive breath odors in the jaundiced patient. "Fetor hepaticus" (said to be a "mousy" odor) was said to suggest perilously impaired liver function. Probably the most frequent olfactory finding in certain jaundiced patients is the "spoiled fruit" aroma that betrays recent ingestion of alcohol. Everyone has encountered more than a few patients who deny having imbibed alcohol, yet contradictorily reek.

> ## *"All icterus is not of the same hue."*

It is important in the physical examination of the jaundiced patient to search for manifestations of antecedent liver disease. One should look for spider nevi, evidence of fluid retention and ascites, and signs of portal hypertension, notably distended veins on the abdominal wall (see Chapter 11, "Ascites"). One should also look for signs of nutritional deficiency in the membranes of the mouth and on the surface of the tongue. In the skin one looks for scratch marks, suggesting pruritus, and for multiple puncture sites on the arms, suggesting the use of illicit drugs.

The size and character of the liver, if it is not obscured by an unduly heavy panniculus or by ascites, may give clues to the duration of liver disease. Inability to detect by palpation or percussion an enlarged liver may mean that the liver is normal or shrunken. An enlarged, very tender liver suggests that the organ has become swollen only recently, as by passive hyperemia or acute inflammation. The liver of a patient with extrahepatic jaundice, because of engorged bile ducts, is almost always palpably enlarged. A large, fat-laden liver is usually not tender. Hard, gross nodularity indicates neoplasia.

Jaundice combined with a palpable, distended gallbladder conforms to Courvoisier's law and points to an obstructive carcinoma at or near the head of the pancreas. Obstructive jaundice due to stone or intrahepatic cholestasis may be attended by an enlarged, tender liver, but not by a palpable gallbladder. A palpable midepigastric mass in a jaundiced patient suspected of harboring pancreatic carcinoma is almost certainly metastatic tumor in liver or omentum and not the primary tumor in the pancreas.

"Courvoisier's law is still in effect and is still valuable."

Despite the diagnostic significance and the important clinical implications of a palpable distended gallbladder, it is common experience that many distended gallbladders escape detection on physical examination of the abdomen. Particularly frustrating is a poorly relaxed abdominal wall. Physicians of earlier years, when encountering this problem, would on occasion resort to a maneuver worth noting in passing. By re-examining the abdomen with the patient immersed in a bathtub filled with tolerably hot water, they found that a distended gallbladder not otherwise palpable could sometimes be felt.

Illustrative Case

A 66-year-old man was admitted to the hospital because of abdominal pain and jaundice. He had had no symptoms suggestive of biliary tract disease until 5 months earlier when he suffered acute, severe upper abdominal pain, became jaundiced almost immediately, and was hospitalized within 24 hours. At that time, examination disclosed an elevated temperature and a tender, right upper abdominal mass interpreted as a tense, inflamed gallbladder. Endoscopic retrograde cholangiopancreatography (ERCP) shortly after admission showed a subtractive defect, thought to represent an impacted stone, in the distal common bile duct. A 1-cm endoscopic sphincterotomy was done, but abdominal pain and fever persisted. Because of this, along with concern about the right upper abdominal mass, the patient was submitted to surgical exploration. This revealed a subhepatic abscess adjacent to a perforated gallbladder and impinging on the anterior wall of the stomach. The gallbladder contained a number of small stones. The abscess was drained and antibiotics were administered. The elevated levels of serum bilirubin, alkaline phosphatase, and aminotransferase activity returned to normal. Repeated cholangiography was reported to show "clearing of any defects in the common bile duct."

The patient seemed to be recovering when, after 4 months, he required readmission to the hospital because of chills, fever, jaundice, and marked weakness. Total serum bilirubin was 3.6 mg per deciliter, alkaline phosphatase was 200 units, and aspartate aminotransferase was 179 units. Blood cultures yielded growth of *Klebsiella pneumoniae* and *Escherichia coli*. Intensive antibiotic therapy led to subsidence of pain and fever. ERCP showed a normal common bile duct. Computed tomography (CT) scans of the liver disclosed no abnormalities; in these images the common bile duct appeared of normal caliber. After 16 days of antibiotic therapy, the serum bilirubin and alkaline phosphatase reverted to nearly normal levels.

Again the patient did fairly well. However, a month later following a heavy meal, he once more suffered acute pain in the epigastrium and right upper abdomen without radiation to the back. Again, he had fever, chills, dark urine, and yellowing of the eyes. This recurrence of symptoms led to the patient's re-admission.

Physical examination was essentially unremarkable except for slight icterus and a temperature of 100.4°F. The white blood cell count was 4,200 cells per milimeter^3, the total serum bilirubin was 3.3 mg per deciliter, and the serum alkaline phosphatase was 114 units. The values for serum aminotransferase, amylase, and lipase activities were normal. Ultrasonography of the right upper abdomen showed no dilated ducts but did suggest slight prominence in the head of the pancreas. ERCP showed a tight stricture of the common bile duct, 1 cm in length, just above the ampulla. No subtractive defects were evident in the common bile duct, and the intrahepatic ducts appeared normal. The narrowed segment in the common bile duct was dilated with an endoscopically guided balloon. Two days later the serum bilirubin was 1.3 mg per deciliter and the serum alkaline phosphatase was 111 units; aminotransferase activities were within normal limits.

At follow-up examination 12 months later, the patient stated that he had remained well and free of recurring abdominal pain, fever, and jaundice. Laboratory values were essentially normal. ERCP was done, with selective cannulation of the bile ducts. Instillation of contrast medium outlined extra- and intrahepatic ducts of normal caliber; there was no evidence of stricture or stones. The contrast material was seen to flow unimpeded from the ducts into the duodenum.

Comment. The clinical situation described here illustrates some of the multiple factors that require consideration and some of the complexities that challenge the clinician who seeks to fathom the nature of disorder in a jaundiced patient.

In keeping with the intent and focus of this volume (see Preface), the discussion that preceded the case presentation concentrated on the diagnostic clues that may be gleaned from a careful analysis of the clinical features in a given patient presenting with jaundice. Although detailed descriptions of ancillary biochemical analysis of urine and serum, imaging techniques, and endoscopic procedures were omitted purposely from the preliminary review, it is stressed that the selective use of these special tests to confirm, extend, modify, or negate impressions drawn from clinical assessment is standard practice and of indisputable value. All the more is this the case when the clinical findings point to cholestasis and extrahepatic obstruction looms as a prominent consideration. In such situations, ancillary diagnostic procedures are indispensable if a definitive diagnosis is to be made.

The principal studies employed today to help substantiate or, if need be, modify the clinical impression involve certain biochemical analyses of serum and urine, imaging techniques, and endoscopic procedures. Discussion of all of these and their uses is beyond the scope of this volume. Brief comment is in order, however, with respect to the roles of these studies in distinguishing between hepatocellular and extrahepatic jaundice, so often a challenge with which the clinician must contend.

Laboratory studies ordinarily resorted to in such situations involve measurement of bilirubin in the serum and urine and assay of the activities of alkaline phosphatase and the aminotransferases in the serum. Elevation of serum bilirubin, principally of the direct-reacting fraction, and of serum alkaline phosphatase, with only slight, if any, increase in activity of the aminotransferases, would suggest cholestasis; elevation in the serum of bilirubin and of aminotransferase activities, with slight or no rise in alkaline phosphatase activity, would support hepatocellular jaundice.

Should there be reason from the clinical assessment to suspect that the jaundice may be arising from pancreatic disease compressing the bile duct and obstructing flow within it, serum amylase and lipase activities would doubtless be measured as well as the level of one of the tumor markers, (e.g., CA19-9 and carcinoembryonic antigen [CEA]).

Imaging procedures presently employed to help identify or exclude extrahepatic obstructive causes for jaundice are abdominal ultrasonography (being extended presently to operative and endoscopic sonography) and computed contrast-enhanced tomography. *Ultrasonography* has the advantage of being noninvasive and is an effective means of delineating the gallbladder and the major extrahepatic bile ducts. Demonstration by this method of gallstones in the gallbladder or the common bile duct, along with evident dilatation of the intrahepatic and extrahepatic bile ducts, would provide strong evidence of underlying calculous obstruction as the cause for the jaundice.

Computed tomography is a more costly study and is attended by radiation exposure. It is a useful means of demonstrating dilated intrahepatic bile ducts suggestive of biliary obstruction and of masses within the liver, but its most valuable application in cases of possible obstructive jaundice is to outline the pancreas and the structures adjacent to it.

Direct opacification of the biliary and pancreatic ducts may be accomplished in retrograde fashion through endoscopically guided introduction of a catheter into the papilla of Vater and then injection of contrast material into the biliary and pancreatic ductal systems (*ERCP*). Ductal opacification may also be secured by the antegrade introduction of contrast material through a catheter placed percutaneously and transhepatically into the biliary ductal system (*PTC*). The opacification of the biliary or pancreatic ducts provided by these approaches allows identification of the presence in or around these ducts of actual or potentially obstructive lesions, such as stones, strictures, and tumors.

Direct inspection of the bile and pancreatic ducts (*cholangioscopy* and *pancreoscopy*) is possible by the use of a "daughter" endoscope placed directly into the bile or pancreatic ducts through a larger housing endoscope.

Endoscopy and its various technical adaptations not only serve to visualize lesions, but also allow biopsies to be taken and bile or pancreatic juice to be aspirated for cytologic examination and assay of tumor marker activity. Through the use of the techniques of endoscopy, therapeutic procedures may additionally be carried out as needed (e.g., sphincterotomy, stone extraction, placement of stents). Utilization of selected objective procedures in helping resolve the intrinsic perplexities of jaundice is demonstrated in the case cited.

The course of events in this rather complex case raises certain challenging questions:

Did the Initial Episode of Pain and Jaundice Actually Mark the Beginning of This Patient's Biliary Tract Disease? The answer to this question is somewhat moot. The initial episode was the first overt clinical expression of underlying biliary tract disease, but the presence of a stone in the common bile duct and the finding of cholelithiasis indicates that calculous biliary tract disease quite likely existed for some time before then.

What Led to the Initial Symptoms? The underlying cause of this event was probably acute cholecystitis initiated by obstruction of the cystic duct by one of the small stones present in the gallbladder. The ensuing acute cholecystitis, in turn, was complicated by the development of empyema, perforation of the gallbladder, and subhepatic abscess. The ductal stone, if it was present then, played no pathogenetic role in the violent inflammatory changes that developed in the gallbladder.

Did the Common Bile Duct Stone Cause the First Episode of Jaundice?   Probably not. The jaundice was more likely related to cholangitis resulting from the cholecystitis and perhaps pressure on the common bile duct by contiguous inflammatory swelling and edema.

Was the First ERCP Necessary?   This is questionable. The patient had been found to have a tense and tender gallbladder, and the physical signs suggested severe, probably suppurative cholecystitis. Abdominal ultrasonography or a CT scan would have been more informative and less hazardous and probably would have disclosed the abscess. ERCP did demonstrate the common bile duct stone (which doubtless would have been found at operative cholangiography, had operation, not been delayed), but the stone in the duct did not play a significant part in the patient's acute problems. It was not in itself responsible for the acute cholecystitis, nor for the jaundice, nor for the complications of perforation and abscess formation.

What Caused the Common Bile Duct Stricture That Later Required Dilation?   Common bile duct strictures occurring in patients who have undergone biliary tract surgery are usually the result of trauma to the duct inflicted by efforts to find and remove intraductal stones. In this case, the stricture may well be attributed to scarring following resolution of the suppurative inflammation or perhaps to scarring at the site of the initial, endoscopic papillotomy. Strictures tend to recur, and it would be advisable to obtain another retrograde cholangiogram after a few months to assess the status of the stricture. Further balloon dilation may be necessary.

To Sum Up

No single problem confronting the clinician exceeds jaundice in the need for correlation of the patient's history and physical examination with data selectively obtained from the laboratory and from imaging procedures. Information obtained directly from the patient permits a discriminating choice of objective tests which, in turn, lead to a correct diagnosis and appropriate treatment. When steps are taken in logical sequence, it is likely that the origin of jaundice can be explained and the underlying cause resolved with the least expenditure of effort, resources, and risk.

References

1. Vennes JA, Bond JH. Approach to the jaundice patient. Gastroenterology 1983; 84:1615–1618.
2. O'Connor KW, Snodgrass PJ, Swonder JS, et al. A blinded prospective study comparing four current non-invasive approaches in the differential diagnosis of medical versus surgical jaundice. Gastroenterology 1983; 84:1498–1504.

3. McNee JW. Jaundice: A review of recent work. Q J Med 1973; 16:190.
4. Oelberg DS, Lester R. Mechanisms of cholestasis. Annu Rev Med 1986; 37:297.
5. Thorpe MEC, Scheuer DJ, Sherlock S. Primary sclerosing cholangitis, the biliary tree and ulcerative colitis. Gut 1967; 8:435–448.
6. Lefkowitch JH, Murtin EE. Primary sclerosing cholangitis. Prog Liver Dis 1986; 8:557–580.

Suggested Reading

Baron RL, Stanley RJ, Lee JKT, et al. A prospective comparison of the evaluation of biliary obstruction using computed tomography and ultrasonography. Radiology 1982; 145:91–98.
Schaffner F, Popper H. Classification and mechanism of cholestasis. A simple algorithm for approaching the problem of cholestasis. In: Wright R, Alberti KGMM, Karran S, Millward-Sadler GH, eds. Liver and biliary disease. Philadelphia: WB Saunders; 1979:315–516.
Scharschmidt BF. Jaundice. In: Sleisenger MH, Fordtran JS, eds. Gastrointestinal disease: Pathophysiology, diagnosis, management. 4th ed. Philadelphia: WB Saunders, 1989:454–467.

ASCITES

John C. Hoefs, M.D.

11

Ascites is peritoneal fluid accumulation due to the displacement of a nearly isosmotic, sodium-containing, proteinaceous fluid into the peritoneal cavity in excess of fluid absorption. To the patient, however, ascites translates as a swollen abdomen and ordinarily it is because of a complaint of swelling of the abdomen that a physician is consulted. Inasmuch as this volume is devoted to digestive system disorders, this chapter deals primarily with ascites. The other major causes of a swollen abdomen are considered only with respect to the features that distinguish them from ascites.

Mechanisms of Ascites Formation

Either protein displacement with secondary sodium retention or primary sodium retention with secondary protein accumulation may lead to ascites. In most cases in which ascites is associated with portal hypertension, primary sodium retention is important in the formation of the fluid collection. When ascites is unrelated to portal hypertension, peritoneal protein accumulation in excess of absorption is prerequisite to the fluid accumulation and secondary sodium retention is required for hemodynamic homeostasis.

Intraperitoneal production of fluid must exceed diaphragmatic fluid absorption for fluid to accumulate as ascites. Net absorption of ascitic fluid occurs only through the diaphragm, where lymphatics open into the peritoneal cavity to allow the net absorption of protein. In all other areas of the peritoneal cavity, hydrostatic and concentration gradients are such that the net movement of protein is only possible into the peritoneal cavity. The volume of fluid formed per unit of time is determined by the net rate of protein transfer into the peritoneal cavity and the amount of dilution required for oncotic-hydrostatic

"To the patient, ascites is a 'swollen abdomen,' and this is the usual presenting complaint."

balance between capillaries and the peritoneal cavity. The net rate of protein transfer is determined by the difference between the amount absorbed through the diaphragm and the amount produced: (1) by specific transfer of protein across the intact capsule and peritoneal membrane on the peritoneal surface of the liver, spleen, and intestines, relative to the specific organ surface permeability and the interstitial fluid to peritoneal cavity hydrostatic gradient; and (2) by fluids leaking through anatomic defects in hollow organs, such as the lymphatics.

"For ascites to develop, intraperitoneal fluid production must exceed diaphragmatic fluid absorption."

When considering hydrostatic gradients, it is important to appreciate that the blood-to-peritoneal-cavity hydrostatic gradient is one of the determinants of dilution of peritoneal fluid and is correlated closely with the A-GRAD (the difference between the serum albumin and ascitic fluid albumin concentrations). However, because there is no major capillary network directly in contact with ascitic fluid, it is the specific organ interstitial fluid-to-peritoneal-cavity hydrostatic gradients (G) acting on a specific organ surface membrane permeability (P) that are important in protein transfer (rate of protein transfer = $P \times G$). Furthermore, the interstitial fluid of the intestines and ascitic fluid have the same hydrostatic and oncotic pressures (hydrostatic gradient = 0) unless the lymphatic drainage from the intestine is blocked. Thus, in most of the disorders that evoke ascites, there are no gradients from the intestinal interstitial compartment to ascitic fluid that would contribute to net transfer of protein into the peritoneal cavity, even in the presence of portal hypertension or increased intestinal peritoneal membrane permeability. Alterations that cause intestinal lymphatic outflow obstruction, such as those that occur with peritoneal carcinomatosis and tuberculosis, may create a hydrostatic gradient not normally present. The latter will increase protein transfer into the peritoneal cavity in the absence of increased permeability.

Abnormalities in the diaphragmatic absorption of peritoneal fluid are thought to be relatively uncommon. In contrast, increased production of fluid is common to nearly all the disorders that may give rise to ascites (Table 11–1). In situations marked by portal hypertension, congestion of the liver increases the transfer of protein across the liver capsule into the peritoneal cavity. Here the transferred proteins are markedly diluted as a result of low serum oncotic pressure and portal hypertension. Both hepatic congestion and dilution are important in determining the amount of fluid formed. Thus, ascites is rare in patients with portal hypertension without liver congestion (e.g., idiopathic portal hypertension). Infinite dilution without significant increase in the rate of protein transfer into the peritoneal cavity is the major factor in oncotic ascites. Other causes of ascites that are not associated with portal hypertension act primarily through increased rate of protein transfer into the peritoneal cavity mediated through a hollow organ leak, increased peritoneal membrane permeability, or intestinal interstitial fluid hypertension secondary to blocked intestinal lymphatics. Often, multiple abnormalities are present.

Disorders Associated With Ascites

Ascites appearing for the first time can be caused by a variety of disorders (Table 11–2). These may be classified into two main groups: (1) those associated with portal hypertension, and (2) those not associated with portal hypertension. Familiarity with the distinctive features of these disorders is helpful in determining the cause of ascites in an individual patient and in differential diagnosis.

> *"Ascites appearing for the first time may be a variety of disorders, of which chronic liver disease is the most common."*

Disorders Associated with Portal Hypertension

Chronic Liver Disease. Ascites related to chronic liver disease (CLD) usually forms late in the course of the disorder, often in response to the following:

TABLE 11-1. Local Mechanisms of Ascites Formation

Cause	Iso-oncotic Absorption Through the Diaphragm	Protein Dilution		Protein Transfer					Hollow Organ Leak
		Serum Oncotic Pressure	Hydrostatic Gradient (Blood to Ascites)	Liver*		Intestine*			
				P	G	P	G		
Associated with portal hypertension									
Cardiac disease	N	N	I	N	I	N	0		–*
Budd-Chiari syndrome	N	N	I	N	I	N	0		–*
Veno-occlusive disease	N	N–D	I	N	I	N	0		–*
Chronic liver disease	N–D	D	I	N	I	N	0		–*
Massive hepatic metastases	N	D	I	N	I	N	0		–*
Hemodialysis	N	N	I	?	I	?	0		–*
Myxedema	N–D	N	I	N	N–I	N	0–I		–(N)
Not associated with portal hypertension									
Peritoneal carcinomatosis	D	D	N	N	N	N	I		±
Inflammation	N–D	D	N	I	N	I	I–0		–
Hollow organ leak	N	N	N	N**	N	I–N**	0		+
Oncotic	N	D	N	N	N	N	0		±
Peritoneal dialysis	D	N	N	?	N	?	0		–

N = normal; 0 = none; D = decreased; I = increased; – = absent; + = present.
*Lymphatic leak was present in 20 percent of patients.
**Inflammatory changes in ascites may increase permeability.

1. An acute flare of the underlying cause of the liver disease (e.g., acute exacerbation of chronic active hepatitis or an alcohol binge by a patient with chronic alcoholic liver disease).
2. Resuscitation for gastrointestinal bleeding.
3. Superimposition of hepatocellular carcinoma.

In questioning the patient, inquiry should scrupulously be made about symptoms suggestive of jaundice or liver disease, the occurrence in the past of liver disease, a family history of liver disease, and the presence of conditions known to predispose to liver disease. Symptoms related to liver disease about which inquiry should especially be made include generalized itching with minimal or secondary skin rash (usually including the palms of the hands and soles of the feet), dark urine and light stools preceding jaundice, right upper quadrant discomfort, and evidence of gastrointestinal bleeding.

Among the conditions known to predispose to CLD are a strong family history, particularly for hemochromatosis; intravenous drug use; substantial alcohol ingestion (usually more than 1 pint per day of hard liquor or its equivalent for at least 10 years); homosexual activity; exposure to certain medications or toxins; an Asian background; and work as a health care provider that involves exposure to blood products.

Chronic liver disease is the most common underlying disorder associated with ascites (Table 11–3). The nature of the liver disease, however, varies in different locales. Alcohol-induced liver disease is the most common form in the United States whereas, worldwide, hepatitis B and C and schistosomiasis are more frequently associated with ascites. Acute and subacute liver disease also may be associated with ascites if the insult is unusually severe. As a rule, deep jaundice is present if this occurs, and the prognosis is poor.

The extra-abdominal, indirect physical signs associated with CLD include palmar erythema, spider angiomas, gynecomastia, alteration in the fingernails ("liver nails"), and clubbing of the distal digits. Testicular atrophy, Dupuytren's contracture and parotid enlargement are commonly noted in alcoholic liver disease; their greater frequency in this disorder, however, may be more closely related to the alcohol intake than to the CLD per se. The microvascular abnormalities (palmar erythema, spider angiomas, clubbing, and gynecomastia) are attributed partly to feminization and are more specific findings in men than in women, except when the abnormalities are well developed and/or numerous. In a man, the presence of even one or two well-developed spider angiomas on the arms is probably indicative of CLD unless there is a family history of these lesions.

Ascites forming for the first time in patients with CLD frequently is associated with jaundice that tends to be milder in degree than with acute hepatic disease. The rise in serum bilirubin concentration produces scleral icterus and yellowness of the mucous membranes. The pigmentary change in these areas is best appreciated in white light and is usually detectable when the serum

TABLE 11–2.   Disorders Associated with Ascites

Disorder	Symptoms	Physical Findings
Intrinsic liver disease	Jaundice* Itching	Jaundice* Liver stigmata* Splenomegaly* Liver—firm/large or small* Abdominal wall collaterals Bruit (with alcoholic hepatitis)
Cardiac disease	Shortness of breath* Dyspnea on exertion* Paroxysmal nocturnal dyspnea	Jugular venous distention* Large liver
Veno-occlusive disease and Budd-Chiari syndrome	Tenderness† RUQ ± jaundice	Large liver Tender liver edge
Chronic Budd-Chiari syndrome with inferior vena caval block above hepatic veins	Tenderness RUQ ± jaundice	Large liver Tender liver edge Dilated veins on back*
Myxedema	Constipation; hoarseness; cold intolerance	Pulse < 60/min* Lateral thinning of eyebrows Increased relaxation phase of reflexes

Malignancy		
Peritoneal carcinomatosis	Anorexia	Firm $(3+-4+)$*
Massive hepatic metastasis	Weight loss	Tenderness RUQ
Hepatocellular carcinoma	Fullness RUQ	Bruit (with hepatocellular carcinoma)
Chronic peritoneal inflammation (tuberculosis, fungus, serositis)	Mild, diffuse abdominal pain	Mild, diffuse tenderness
	Anorexia	Fever
	Night sweats	
	Low-grade fever	
Hollow organ leak		
Infected	Abdominal pain	Abdominal tenderness
	Chills and fever	
Noninfected		
Chemical peritonitis	Abdominal pain	± Mild tenderness
No chemical peritonitis	Abdominal pain	
Oncotic		
Nephrotic	Anasarca	Anasarca*
		Increased blood pressure*
Nutritional	Steatorrhea	Muscle wasting
	Anasarca	Anasarca

*Finding that was pathognomonic or present in more than 90 percent of patients.

†RUQ = right upper quadrant.

TABLE 11–3. Comparative Frequencies of Disorders Associated with Ascites (Initial Episodes) as Encountered in the United States

Disorder	Frequency (%)
Chronic liver disease	83
Malignancy	10
Massive hepatic metastases	3.3
Peritoneal carcinomatosis	6.6
Heart failure	3
Tuberculous	1
Nononcotic nephrogenous	1
Nephrotic	<1
Hollow organ leak	<1
Nontuberculous serositis	<1
Budd-Chiari syndrome and veno-occlusive disease	<1
Chylous	<1
Myxedema	<1

bilirubin is greater than 3 mg per deciliter. The clinical dictum that ascites that forms in the presence of jaundice is due to parenchymal liver disease appears well founded. However, disorders featuring hepatic congestion, such as cardiac disease, Budd-Chiari syndrome, and veno-occlusive disease, are also potential causes.

Examination of the abdomen may disclose a caput medusae, hepatic enlargement or shrinkage, increased firmness of the liver, splenomegaly, hepatic bruit, or a Cruveilhier-Baumgarten murmur. The caput medusae represents extensive shunting from the portal system to the anterior abdominal wall through the umbilical vein. Less than 20 percent of patients with CLD who develop ascites will have this finding, although nearly all will have a prominent venous pattern over the abdomen if the ascites is sufficient to make the abdominal wall tense (Fig. 11–1). A prominent venous pattern on the abdominal wall is nonspecific; it may be seen in disorders not associated with portal hypertension and without collateral circulation. This abnormal abdominal wall venous pattern is most prominent when there is peripheral wasting of muscle and fat. In differentiating visible veins in the abdominal wall from the extensive and prominent abdominal wall collateral veins that develop with portal hypertension, it is helpful to keep in mind that the latter may be felt as well as seen.

Sometimes, particularly in earlier stages or when the abdominal wall still has a fair amount of fat, engorgement of the abdominal veins may be faint. If the abdominal wall is viewed through the red goggles employed by radiologists in pre-image amplifier days to adapt their eyes before conducting a fluoroscopic examination, the veins are much more apparent.

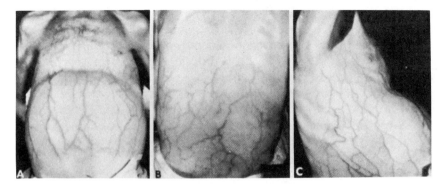

FIGURE 11-1. Prominent veins over the abdomen and back in a man with hepatic cirrhosis and pronounced ascites. A, Anterior view of abdomen; B, back; C, lateral view of abdomen. (Reproduced with permission from Levitt RE, Roth JLA, eds. General Physical Examination. In: Berk JE, Haubrich WS, Kalser MH, Roth JLA, Schaffner F, eds. Bockus Gastroenterology. 4th ed. Philadelphia: WB Saunders, 1985: 262.

The direction of flow in the visible abdominal veins is normally upward in the upper one-third of the abdomen and downward in the lower two-thirds. When the veins are distended because of portal hypertension, the direction of flow is unchanged. When there is an obstruction in the inferior vena cava, however, the direction of flow of the collateral veins in the lower abdomen is reversed.

The size of the liver and its degree of firmness are important to estimate. In disorders productive of ascites that are associated with portal hypertension, the liver may be large or small and, if it can be felt, is usually mildly to moderately firm. A large liver usually indicates an acute or subacute insult, whereas a small one is more compatible with far-advanced cirrhosis. The liver often is difficult to feel in the presence of ascites. This difficulty may be resolved through the use of ballottement, which is a rapid, dipping-inward pressure on the abdominal wall with the tips of the fingers to detect the resistance imparted by the floating liver. Another approach is to re-examine the abdomen after removing 5 to 6 liters of ascitic fluid. The liver still may not be palpable after the fluid has been removed, however, because it is small and tucked up under the rib cage or is normal in size but soft in consistency.

The spleen tends to enlarge in cases of parenchymal liver disease as a consequence of congestion secondary to portal hypertension. Indeed, splenomegaly usually is an indication of appreciable and longstanding portal hypertension. Splenic enlargement develops as a rule at a rate of 1 to 3 cm per year after the portal pressure equals or exceeds 10 mm Hg over the pressure in the inferior vena cava. In cases of acute and subacute hepatic injury, such as alcoholic hepatitis, the spleen may be only mildly enlarged. Approximately 95 percent of cirrhotic patients with well-established disease, particularly cirrhosis of nonalcoholic origin, will exhibit mild to marked splenomegaly. The so-called spleen percussion sign (tympany in the left lateral rib cage over the spleen, changing to dullness on inspiration) is normally positive when the spleen is more than 13 cm in length; the tip of the spleen is usually palpable when splenic length is more than 15 cm.

A hepatic arterial bruit may be heard in cases of alcoholic hepatitis, due to marked arterial flow. A bruit also may be audible when an arteriovenous communication is present, such as occurs with hepatocellular carcinoma. As a general rule, alcoholic hepatitis and hepatocellular cancer may be held to account for 95 percent of hepatic bruits if aortic compression can be ruled out by repositioning of the body. Other arteriovenous communications giving rise to audible bruits are for the most part traumatic in origin (including the traumatic changes imposed by needle aspiration biopsy of the liver). Arteriovenous malformations developing in such conditions as Osler-Weber-Rendu disease may also be attended by a bruit.

The Cruveilhier-Baumgarten murmur is a continuous hum in the midline near the umbilicus resulting from portal hypertension with rapid flow of blood through a patent umbilical vein into the abdominal wall collaterals. Turbulence is produced above the umbilicus as blood traveling caudad in the umbilical vein turns sharply cephalad to feed upper abdominal wall collaterals leading into the internal mammary system. Large abdominal wall venous collaterals typically are present as well. The hum characteristically decreases with deep inspiration and with pressure over the umbilicus.

Acute bacterial peritonitis is present in 15 percent to 25 percent of patients with ascites due to CLD. The peritonitis is frequently asymptomatic or mildly symptomatic and most often is detected early only by paracentesis and examination of the ascitic fluid. At least half of the patients have neither abdominal pain nor fever. Spontaneous bacterial peritonitis, a form marked by the absence of an infected focus or perforation within the peritoneal cavity, accounts for 95 percent of the cases with peritonitis. The clinical course in most untreated patients is characterized by progressive worsening, with the development of diffuse abdominal pain and tenderness, fever, mental confusion, progressive hepatic failure, coagulopathy, renal failure, or gastrointestinal bleeding. Patients with ascites who present with such features, or who develop them subsequently, require paracentesis to determine if peritonitis may be the cause.

Other Disorders Associated With Portal Hypertension.   All of the disorders in this group may have the same clinical features as CLD, except for the peripheral stigmas of liver disease. Mild jaundice is common and may be deep on occasion. Typically the liver is large, 1 + to 2 + in firmness, and often slightly tender.

Cardiac Disease.   Ascites whose genesis is cardiac disease arises from right heart failure due to constrictive disease (e.g., constrictive pericarditis or constrictive cardiomyopathy) or tricuspid insufficiency (either valvular or as a nonspecific response to right ventricular dilatation). Over 85 percent of patients have a dilated heart with secondary tricuspid insufficiency and a history of recurrent congestive heart failure. In addition, the patient will usually describe an increase in symptoms (shortness of breath, orthopnea, paroxysmal nocturnal dyspnea, and ankle swelling) in the period immediately preceding ascites formation. Often the symptoms of heart failure improve as the ascites forms. This is in contradistinction to tense ascites unrelated to cardiac disease, in which many of the same symptoms may be described but only after the ascites and tenseness have developed. Untreated patients with cardiac ascites will display prominent neck veins when sitting at a 90-degree angle, especially if the ascites has been progressively increasing. Jugular venous distention can disappear rapidly with effective therapy for heart failure and may not be present a few hours after admission; the initial examination therefore is critical to the diagnosis. Peripheral dependent edema is characteristic of cardiac ascites, and anasarca may be present as well.

Budd-Chiari Syndrome and Veno-occlusive Disease. Budd-Chiari syndrome and veno-occlusive disease are due to blockage of hepatic venous outflow. When this occurs acutely (e.g., after trauma), jaundice, right upper quadrant abdominal pain, and hepatic failure are features. In contrast, chronic Budd-Chiari syndrome and veno-occlusive disease may present only with ascites. Examination demonstrates hepatomegaly with a 1 + to 2 + firm liver edge, splenomegaly, and evidence of portal hypertension. Chronic Budd-Chiari syndrome may follow the acute variant or, more frequently, may appear insidiously. Myeloproliferative disorders, paroxysmal nocturnal hemoglobinuria, use of birth control pills, and hypercoagulable states are associated with this syndrome. Hepatic tumors in the dome of the liver may also be responsible for the syndrome by compressing hepatic venous outflow. In about half of the patients, the cause is not apparent, but many of these patients are now suspected of having a premyeloproliferative condition. Veno-occlusive disease is uncommon in the United States, except for cases following radiation to the liver (usually greater than 3,000 REM) and bone marrow transplantation.

Chronic Budd-Chiari syndrome originating from inferior vena caval blockage above the entrance of the hepatic veins characteristically causes dilatation of collateral veins over the back as well as the abdomen. Hence, the finding of dilated veins over the back serves as a pathognomonic sign of such blockage in the setting of ascites. The explanation for the prominent back veins lies in the marked interference with blood returning to the heart. An extensive and large collateral flow is required to compensate for the diminished cardiac return in order to maintain systemic hemodynamics. Inasmuch as collaterals can only develop to the mediastinum and the anterior and the posterior abdominal walls, pronounced collateral circulation develops through the vertebral veins leading to dilated paravertebral back veins.

Massive Hepatic Metastasis. One-third of patients with ascites due to malignancy have massive hepatic metastasis. The liver usually is markedly enlarged and very firm. The degree of firmness is generally greater than that in most patients with liver enlargement due to CLD or hepatic congestion and may be so pronounced as to be "rock-hard."

Myxedema. Myxedematous ascites usually is multifactorial but ordinarily is associated with portal hypertension attributed to subclinical cardiac failure. Classic features include hoarse voice, lateral thinning of the eyebrows, dry skin, pulse rate of less than 60 per minute, and mild arterial hypertension. The presence of such signs suggests the diagnosis, and a prolonged relaxation phase of the peripheral nerve reflexes adds confirmatory evidence. Jaundice is rare.

Disorders Not Associated with Portal Hypertension

In general, these disorders are notable clinically for the absence of features commonly found in disorders associated with portal hypertension (i.e., peripheral stigmas of cirrhotic liver disease, a firm liver, splenomegaly, and jugular vein distention). Jaundice also is uncommon unless the biliary system is obstructed, as by pancreatic cancer.

Peritoneal Carcinomatosis. Ascites that forms in the presence of a known primary or metastatic cancer is likely to be due to cancer. Two-thirds of patients with ascites due to cancer have peritoneal carcinomatosis. With an established cancer known to have metastasized elsewhere, peritoneal carcinomastosis is likely if ascites is evident and the liver is not firm and enlarged. Abdominal masses occasionally may be palpable, and sometimes distended bowel due to partial bowel obstruction may be readily observed. In a patient not known to have cancer, the finding of a mass elsewhere or of blood in the stool suggests the possibility that fluid accumulation in the peritoneal cavity is the result of peritoneal carcinomatosis.

Oncotic Ascites. Oncotic ascites is due to a very low serum colloid osmotic pressure (10 to 12 mm Hg) resulting from protein loss or malnutrition. In the United States, the most common cause of oncotic ascites is the nephrotic syndrome, but a protein-losing gastroenteropathy and kwashiorkor should also be considered in some cases. The hallmark of this variety of ascites is a very low serum albumin level (less than 1.5 g per deciliter), producing anasarca and dependent edema. The nephrotic syndrome is associated with hypertension, proteinuria, and a hypercoagulable state. Associated nutritional deficiencies may promote marked muscle wasting.

Hollow Organ Leak. Leakage of fluid from any hollow organ may result in ascites. If the fluid leaking from the hollow structure is infected, the presentation is apt to be that of acute peritonitis, but such instances are rare. Leakage of sterile fluid from the pancreatic duct, the biliary ducts, or the gut may excite a chemical peritonitis with polymorphonuclear response in the peritoneal fluid.

Pancreatic ascites, seen most often in alcohol abusers, ensues from rupture into the peritoneal cavity of a pseudocyst or a pancreatic duct. An asymptomatic chemical peritonitis usually is present in these cases, with less than half of the patients describing pain or displaying the clinical features of pancreatitis. Occasionally, an abdominal pseudocyst may be felt.

A lymphatic leak usually is asymptomatic. If the leakage is from lacteals, the ascitic fluid appears chylous (white and opaque, like milk). Chylous ascites frequently follows trauma (e.g., a motor vehicle accident or an operation). Spontaneous chylous ascites usually is due to blockage by a tumor (often lymphoma) or tuberculosis at the entrance of the left thoracic duct into the left subclavian vein.

Chronic Inflammatory Ascites.   Chronic serositis or peritonitis may be associated with mild, diffuse abdominal pain. Ordinarily, however, these conditions are not attended by symptoms related to the abdomen or by abnormal findings on abdominal examination. In this regard, chronic inflammatory ascites is similar to spontaneous or secondary infection of cirrhotic ascites. The detection on examination of diffuse peritoneal tenderness or muscle guarding should be taken seriously, particularly if the tenderness is present in the absence of tense ascites or if it remains after tense ascites is decompressed.

Chronic peritonitis with a lymphocytic cellular response in the ascitic fluid most often proves to be tuberculous. A similar response may also be found, however, when the infectious agent is *Chlamydia* or a fungus. In these patients, a low-grade fever often is present, and features of chronic disease, such as anorexia and profound muscle wasting, may be noted. Patients actually may lose weight as the ascites increases as a consequence of inadequate food intake and the increased catabolism of inflammation.

Serositis with a polymorphonuclear cellular reaction in the peritoneal fluid occurs at times with rheumatic diseases, particularly rheumatoid arthritis associated with rheumatoid nodules, and systemic lupus erythematosus. Ascites accompanying eosinophilic gastroenteritis will show a predominance of eosinophils.

Clinical Features

The peritoneal cavity is a potential space that normally contains less than 25 ml of fluid. Any amount greater than this is abnormal, but clinical symptoms ordinarily are not manifest when the volume of fluid is less than 2,000 ml. If untreated, ascites usually increases fairly rapidly and tends to become massive before a new steady state between formation and absorption is obtained.

Uninhibited ascitic fluid accumulation causes the abdomen to swell and body weight to increase over a period of a few weeks.

Suspicion of ascites would be aroused when (1) abdominal swelling and weight gain are noted, (2) nonspecific complaints are presented that could be explained by ascites, or (3) a condition that is associated with ascites is thought to be present. In such circumstances the interrogation of the patient must be firmly rooted in a knowledge of the pathophysiology of ascites and a full appreciation of the inherent limitations of a subjective history.

"Clinical symptoms are not ordinarily manifest when the volume of fluid is less than 200 ml."

History

Viewed in a general way, history taking is affected, among other things, by cultural factors, language barriers, and the relative intelligence, motivation, denial, and articulateness of the patient (see Chapter 1, "History Taking: The Art of Dialogue"). Basically, the greater the number of barriers to communication and the less the spontaneity of response, the lower the credence that can be given to the history. A history characterized by classic complaints that are presented with little or no prompting is a powerful tool in the clinical evaluation of the patient. A history that succeeds in eliciting the classic features of the illness only in response to specific questions is less valuable. Of dubious value is a history in which nonclassic clinical features are described, and even then only with much prompting. Such a history should be given weight only if documented by other sources or supported by confirmatory evidence derived from physical examination.

The specific complaints of most patients presenting with ascites are abdominal swelling, weight gain over a period of a few days to weeks, and concomitant loss of muscle mass from the extremities and chest. In some cases of ascites, notably those secondary to tuberculosis or peritoneal carcinomatosis, the combination of profound anorexia and increased catabolism may result in weight loss instead of gain as the ascites increases. When the peritoneal fluid causes the abdomen to become tense, other problems may emerge, such as shortness of breath, paroxysmal nocturnal dyspnea, abdominal fullness, abdominal discomfort, and early satiety. Ankle edema may develop consequent to low serum oncotic pressure and increased pressure in the inferior vena cava, particularly when there is portal hypertension and the serum albumin concentration is less than 2.5 g per deciliter. Occasionally, anasarca and pleural effusions evolve secondary to sodium retention. The protruding abdomen, swollen by the fluid sequestered in the peritoneal cavity, may affect stability and cause the patient to fall when walking.

When information is not spontaneously offered by the patient, certain questions should be posed directly. These are aimed at determining what actually happened in terms of the patient's experience. Once the major features of the history are obtained, it is advisable to re-question the patient to confirm that the data recorded are consistent and accurate. Typical questions that the physician should ask include the following:

Has weight been gained? If so, how much? And over what period of time?
Did weight increase and then decrease? Has it happened before? What was the cause?
What parts of the body were swollen? The whole body? The legs? Only the abdomen?
What other symptoms occurred? Was there shortness of breath, or paroxysms of shortness of breath, during sleeping hours? Has there been wasting of the arms and legs? Has appetite been lost? (see Chapter 13, "Anorexia").
Has there been a reduction in strength?

If the patient has noted that his or her abdomen was swollen, questioning would focus on details:

Is the swelling diffuse? Over what period of time did it develop? How was it noted?
Did the patient's pants or dresses become tight? Was it found necessary to loosen the belt a notch or two?
Have the feet been swollen? If so, did they swell before or after the abdomen began to swell?
Have menstrual periods ceased? Have there been symptoms similar to those in early pregnancy?
Is the swelling more prominent in the lower abdomen? If the abdominal swelling has been associated with other problems, what was the order of appearance?
Has there been abdominal discomfort or pain? Any nausea or vomiting?

Should the answers to the foregoing questions encourage suspicion of ascites, further questioning would be directed at determining the possible underlying cause:

Is there a history of liver disease? Has intake of alcohol been excessive? Have any parenteral injections been received? Is there a family history of liver disease? Has the urine darkened? Has yellowing of the eyes been noted?
Has there been any right upper quadrant discomfort? Is there a cardiac history? Or a condition that would dispose to Budd-Chiari syndrome or veno-occlusive disease?
Is there a history of malignancy? Or pancreatitis? Or tuberculosis?
What is the patient's ethnic background? What is his or her travel experience?
Are there any kidney problems or known diabetes mellitus? Has the patient been taking thyroid medication or have a history of thyroid disease?
Have there been chills and fever?

When a patient presents with such nonspecific complaints as "indigestion," wasting of the arms and legs, anorexia, or early satiety, ascites may be the cause, although it is unusual for the patient not to have noticed coexistent or antecedent abdominal swelling. Similarly, patients who present with jaundice, or are found to have hepatomegaly, not infrequently have ascites and should be questioned accordingly. Denial of ascites, even when present, is frequent in alcoholics.

Should physical examination disclose ascites that was not anticipated from the history obtained, the patient should be questioned again in detail regarding such items as weight gain, muscle wasting, and progressive swelling of the abdomen.

Physical Findings

Physical examination is of paramount importance in establishing the presence of ascites and in the search for the factors responsible for the condition. If the amount of fluid is small, its presence may not be detected on physical examination. The most sensitive sign is bilateral flank dullness and the most specific sign is shifting dullness. Both are likely to be present when there is more than 1,500 ml of fluid in the peritoneal cavity. Percussion over the normal intestine-filled abdomen gives a widely distributed tympanitic note. When ascites is present, the gas-containing intestines float to the top of the abdominal cavity, and the fluid is displaced to the sides. The laterally dispersed fluid gives a dull note on percussion, commonly described as "coronal" dullness. This crown-like, bilateral flank dullness imparted by the ascitic fluid may be elicited by soft percussion in a patient of normal weight and by hard percussion in an obese patient. Unilateral flank dullness caused by a local mass or an enlarged abdominal organ should be distinguished from the bilateral and symmetric dullness on percussion when fluid occupies both flank areas.

> *"If the amount of fluid is small, its presence may not be detected by physical examination."*

A change in the percussion note from dull, when the patient is supine, to tympanitic over the superior flank, when the patient turns on one side or the other, denotes fluid movement and constitutes "shifting" dullness. This phenomenon is akin to the way in which residual air in a water-filled balloon remains superior as the balloon is rotated. The same concept pertains to the "puddle sign," a physical finding that may be elicited when the patient is placed on all fours and the midabdomen is percussed in its most dependent position, where fluid in the abdomen will gravitate. Using this maneuver, percussion dullness may be obtained with as little as 300 ml of fluid in the peritoneal cavity.

A fluid wave is another classic sign found in the presence of ascites. The value of this sign is limited, however, because it is present only when the volume of fluid is large enough to render the abdominal wall tense. A gentle tap on one side produces a compression wave that can be felt on the other side. To avoid misinterpretation, however, "jiggling" of the abdominal wall produced by the tap must be eliminated. This commonly is accomplished by having another person interpose the side of his or her hand on the abdomen between the examiner's hands. For the experienced clinician, however, this maneuver is ordinarily unnecessary.

Pedal edema and pleural effusions frequently are found in patients with ascites, related in large part to sodium retention. Peripheral muscle wasting and loss of fat are commonplace, as are stigmas such as palmar erythema and spider nevi in patients with CLD. In patients with a swollen abdomen without evidence of primary hepatic disease, findings such as prominent jugular veins and demonstrable hepatojugular reflux (indicative of congestive heart failure), venous collaterals over the back, signs of myxedema, or the finding of lesions compatible with cancer increase the likelihood that the abdominal distention is due to fluid sequestration in the peritoneal cavity.

Differential Diagnosis

The physical examination is of fundamental importance in the differential diagnosis. Certain key findings that are helpful in this regard are noted in Table 11–4. Of central importance is the detection of certain distinctive signs that suggest chronic or subacute liver disease: peripheral liver stigmas (spider nevi, liver palms, clubbing), jaundice, a firm and/or enlarged liver, and a palpable spleen. Such signs will be evident in the vast majority of patients with underlying liver disease. When ascites is massive or when the abdomen is tense and protruding, as much as 5 to 6 liters of fluid may have to be removed to fully assess liver firmness and size, spleen size, and other abdominal masses.

Patients with disorders other than parenchymal liver disease that are associated with portal hypertension and may be attended by ascites may have a firm, enlarged liver, splenomegaly, and mild icterus. Only rarely, however, do such patients manifest peripheral liver stigmas or a small, contracted liver. As already noted, certain other findings on physical examination are of decided value in the differential diagnosis; namely, dilated neck veins (almost invariably found in patients with cardiac ascites) and dilated paravertebral veins over the back (a characteristic of chronic Budd-Chiari syndrome with blockage of the inferior vena cava above the entry of the hepatic veins).

Distended veins in the abdominal wall may be seen with any of the causes for ascites associated with portal hypertension (Figure 11–1). They must be distinguished, however, from the abdominal veins that may be evident when

TABLE 11-4. Differential Diagnosis of Ascites

	Weight Gain	Abdominal Swelling	Bilateral Flank Dullness	Shifting Dullness	Central Tympany
Ascites	Few days to 2 months	General	+	+	+
Pregnancy	Months (3–9)	Hypogastric	–	–	–
Abdominal tumor or cyst	Months (2+)	General or local	–	–	–
Abdominal wall hematoma	1 day to months	Local	–	–	±
Pelvic cyst	Months (4+)	General or hypogastric	–	–	–
Obesity	Months (4+)	General	–	±	+
Intestinal gaseous distention	None	General	–	–	+

TABLE 11-5. Diagnostic Value of Ascitic Fluid Analysis

Test	Indicative of:	Accuracy (%)*
A-GRAD†(>1.1 g/dl)	Portal hypertension	98
Polymorphonuclear cells > 250/mm³	Acute peritonitis	99
Polymorphonuclear cells > 250/mm³ ascites LDH > serum LDH glucose < 50 mg/dl	Secondary severe acute peritonitis (100% sensitive for perforation)	91
Lymphocytes > 500/mm³	Chronic peritonitis or lymphoma	98
Total protein concentration (with A-GRAD > 1.1 g/dl) <1.0 g/dl 1.1-2.0 g/dl > 2.0 g/dl	Tendency for spontaneous bacterial peritonitis	30–50‡ 10–15‡ <5‡
Cytology	Peritoneal carcinomatosis	99
Bacterial culture	Bacterial infection	97
Culture for *Mycobacterium tuberculosis*	Tuberculosis	96
Bilirubin, amylase, creatinine, triglyceride in ascites = 2× serum	Hollow organ leak	99

*Percentage of true positives and true negatives.
†Serum-to-ascites albumin concentration gradient.
‡Percentage of patients who have or who will develop spontaneous bacterial peritonitis during hospital admission.

ascites unassociated with portal hypertension produces a tense abdomen. The latter almost totally disappear after removal of the ascitic fluid, whereas those related to portal hypertension are little altered. Also, as noted earlier, the prominent abdominal veins accompanying portal hypertension can often be felt as well as seen.

Abdominal prominence is a highlight of other conditions, and because of this feature alone they may simulate ascites. Salient aspects that help distinguish ascites from these simulating conditions are listed in Table 11–5. In a woman of childbearing age, pregnancy should be considered when there is weight gain and abdominal protuberance. Differential distinctions include the tendency for the swelling to be hypogastric, the cessation of menstrual periods, and the presence of symptoms classically associated with early pregnancy. The abdominal swelling and weight gain of pregnancy are also slower than in most patients with ascites of recent onset.

A large abdominal or pelvic mass may resemble ascites. Although solid tumors can occasionally do this, abdominal and pelvic cysts do so more often. As with pregnancy, weight gain and protuberance evolve much more slowly. A person with obvious abdominal swelling of more than 2 years is highly unlikely to have ascites; yet this is common in patients with a massive ovarian cyst. An abdominal wall hematoma may resemble ascites occasionally. The fairly rapid appearance of hematoma in the setting of trauma and its development in a patient taking an anticoagulant drug are helpful distinguishing features.

Obese patients with a prominent abdomen ("beer belly") not uncommonly are thought to have ascites. The physical findings serve to differentiate the two conditions, although a fat-laden abdomen may sometimes exhibit shifting dullness. Gaseous distention of the bowel can cause abdominal protuberance, but it is not associated with weight gain. Furthermore, it tends to be intermittent (day-to-day) over a period of years and may be accompanied by other gastrointestinal symptoms. A helpful maneuver in such instances is to lift up the abdomen with both hands as the patient lies on his or her side. If fluid is present, the abdomen will feel heavy; with gas or fat, the abdomen will be comparatively lighter and easier to lift.

Confirmation of Diagnosis

The first two steps in the evaluation of patients in whom ascites is suspected are (1) to prove that ascites is present, and then (2) to consider the relative likelihood of its several causes. With respect to the latter, the attentive clinician will not stray far from the most frequent cause within his or her population of patients. For example, tuberculous ascites may be infrequent in the general population, but its occurrence rate in a tuberculosis sanatorium would be distinctly higher. Similarly, ascites appearing for the first time that is attended by atypical features more likely represents a common cause of ascites with unusual expressions rather than a rare disorder.

Today, the presence or absence of ascites is confirmed most easily and with least risk by abdominal ultrasonography. This examination will also demonstrate the best site to introduce an aspirating needle. When the presence of ascites is quite obvious from the history and physical findings, however, confirmation may be made by a diagnostic peritoneal tap. This less costly and simple procedure at the same time allows aspiration of a sample of the ascitic fluid for analytical studies.

"Ascites is confirmed most easily and with least risk by ultrasonography; however, when it is clinically obvious, ascites may be confirmed by peritoneal tap and analytic studies of the fluid."

The peritoneal tap may be regarded as an extension of the physical examination. It should be accompanied by the simultaneous withdrawal of blood for the same tests to be performed on the ascitic fluid (see Table 11–5). The results obtained will (1) confirm the presence or absence of portal hypertension from the difference between the serum and ascites albumin concentrations; (2) confirm the presence of acute or chronic peritonitis from the cell count and differential analysis; (3) determine the presence of increased metabolic activity; (4) identify spontaneous bacterial peritonitis; (5) provide evidence supportive of hollow organ leak; (6) indicate malignancy from the cytologic findings and, occasionally, from the grossly bloody appearance of the fluid; and (7) indicate the presence of infection from smear and culture of the aspirate.

Illustrative Case

A 55-year-old postmenopausal woman was admitted because of weakness for 6 weeks and increasing abdominal girth for the last 3 weeks. Originally her weight had increased to 136 pounds, but recently her weight fell to below her usual weight of 123 pounds. Her arms and legs had thinned notably. The patient had experienced some night sweats without chills or fever, and she had noted some shortness of breath when supine during the 2 days before admission. There was no history of abdominal pain, peripheral edema, jaundice, excessive alcohol intake, transfusions, intravenous drug abuse, medication use, or previous chronic liver disease or tuberculosis. Constipation, hoarseness, and hypertension were all denied. On examination, the diaphragms were elevated on percussion, and a few dry rales were heard in the base of the right lung. The abdomen was protuberant and displayed a prominent venous pattern. Flank dullness and shifting dullness were elicited. All other physical findings were unremarkable.

Ultrasonography confirmed the presence of ascites. A 20-gauge needle was hence introduced into the peritoneal cavity at a point in the midline below the umbilicus, hence with the patient in the right lateral recumbent position. This yielded 100 ml of thick, slightly opaque fluid that formed a clot in the nonanticoagulant tube. A serum sample was obtained simultaneously for albumin, total protein, lactic dehydrogenase, glucose, and amylase assays. A request was made for the ascitic fluid to be examined for cell count and differential analysis, culture for bacteria, Gram stain, stain for acid-fast bacilli, cytologic examination, and measurement of albumin, total protein, lactic dehydrogenase, glucose and amylase levels. The results of these examinations are shown in Table 11–6.

Comment. The history in this case is highlighted by abdominal protuberance accompanied by weight gain and then loss. If the weight gain had not been documented, other causes for a swollen abdomen would have had to be considered. However, the patient is postmenopausal and does not have other gastrointestinal symptoms, and tissue-wasting as evidenced by the thinning of the arms and legs would explain weight loss even as fluid accumulated in the abdomen. Based on these features and the supporting signs on physical

TABLE 11–6.   Results of Tests (Illustrative Case)

Test	Ascitic Fluid	Serum
Cell count/mm³		
RBC	90	
WBC	1330*	
Albumin (g/dl)	2.2	2.8 (A-GRAD† = 0.6)
Total protein (g/dl)	4.2	5.7
Amylase (U/liter)	30	40
LDH (IU/liter)	215	189
Glucose (mg/dl)	83	100
Oncotic pressure (mm Hg)	12.3	18.6 (Gr = 6.3)
Gram stain	–	
Culture	–	
Acid-fast bacilli	–	
Cytology	–	

*P = 25%, L = 72%, M = 3%
†Serum-to-ascites albumin concentration gradient.
RBC = red blood cell; WBC = white blood cell; P = polymorphonuclear cells; L = lymphocytes; M = mononuclear cells; Gr = gradient; – = negative.

examination, ascites would seem to be the most likely cause for the abdominal prominence.

The lack of a history of liver disease or of exposure to situations associated with chronic liver disease diminishes the likelihood of hepatic derangement as the basis of the ascites, despite its statistical frequency. In addition, ascites associated with liver disease usually has an inciting event that frequently is associated with jaundice; namely, an acute flare of the basic hepatic injury, variceal bleeding necessitating resuscitative measures, or the development of hepatocellular carcinoma. None of these was evident in this patient. Hence, causes for ascites other than chronic liver disease is the primary consideration.

Second to chronic liver disease in order of frequency among the causes for ascites is malignancy, and in half of the patients with cancerous ascites the accumulation of peritoneal fluid is the first clinical manifestation. Malignant tumors contribute to ascites formation in several ways, including massive hepatic metastasis, peritoneal carcinomatosis, lymphatic flow blockage, and hepatic vein obstruction (Budd-Chiari syndrome). The history given by this patient of weight loss as the ascitic fluid increased in volume supported the possibility of underlying cancer. On the other hand, the absence of a firm, palpable liver militates against massive hepatic metastases, and a chylous appearance of the ascites was not found. Nevertheless, peritoneal carcinomatosis remains a distinct possibility.

Congestive heart failure is another consideration. However, in this patient there is no history of cardiac disease previous to the abdominal swelling, and shortness of breath while she was supine occurred only when the amount of fluid became pronounced. In addition, shortness of breath and exertional dyspnea often precede the development of ascites when the latter is related to cardiac failure, and neither of these occurred in this patient.

There is no history of trauma that might dispose to Budd-Chiari syndrome. Similarly, there was no previous exposure to radiation or ingestion of agents capable of causing veno-occlusive disease. Also, the liver was not palpably enlarged.

Tuberculous ascites requires consideration, even though this is relatively uncommon in the United States. Weighing against this possibility is the lack of symptoms or signs that would point to this disorder, except perhaps for the night sweats. Other possible causes of ascites are not only infrequent in general but also are highly unlikely in this case. Oncotic-related ascites generally is attended by a history of anasarca, and nephrogenous ascites is associated with established chronic or acute renal failure, neither of which obtained here. No symptoms were described and no signs were evident that might suggest myxedematous ascites. Lymphatic leak and pancreatic leakage cannot be excluded with certainty; however, the history and physical findings provide no support for these entities.

The studies made on the ascitic fluid and serum (see Table 11–6) showed that the A-GRAD was narrow, a finding consistent with the absence of portal hypertension. This virtually rules out the category of diseases associated with portal hypertension, including chronic liver disease, and confirms the clinical impression of a cause not associated with portal hypertension. The elevated white blood cell count with a predominance of lymphocytes is consistent with tuberculosis. The mild consumption of glucose and the increase in lactic dehydrogenase activity are also compatible with this disease. The low amylase activity excludes fairly well a pancreatic origin for the ascites. Although peritoneal carcinomatosis occasionally is accompanied by an increased white blood cell count and frequently shows mild metabolic activity in the ascitic fluid, both of which were observed in this patient, the negative cytologic examination weighs against peritoneal carcinomatosis. Stain of the sediment for acid-fast bacilli was negative, but this is common even when tuberculous peritonitis is present.

Peritoneoscopy showed studding of the peritoneum with nodules larger than 2 mm in diameter, and granulomas were evident on biopsy. Within 2 weeks, the cultures of the ascitic fluid and the peritoneal biopsy both disclosed mycobacteria by the DNA hybridization technique. Antituberculous medication was started on the day that peritoneoscopy was done. Within a week, the patient's temperature was normal and the ascites ultimately resolved.

To Sum Up

Ascites results when intraperitoneal fluid production exceeds fluid absorption. A host of conditions may lead to ascites as a consequence of their effect on any of the basic factors determining fluid accumulation in the peritoneal cavity.

A detailed history firmly rooted in knowledge of the pathophysiology of ascites is fundamental to its clinical evaluation. Based on the history, physical examination complemented by ultrasonography of the abdomen or a diagnostic peritoneal tap will confirm the existence of ascites. Examinations made on aspirated ascitic fluid may provide helpful clues to its possible cause.

Suggested Reading

Hoefs JC. Serum concentration and portal pressure determines the ascitic fluid protein concentration in patients with chronic liver disease. J Lab Clin Med 1983; 102:260–273.

Hoefs JC, Runyon B. Spontaneous bacterial peritonitis. Disease-A-Month 1985; 31:3–48.

Hoefs JC. Diagnostic paracentesis: A potent clinical tool. [Editorial] Gastroenterology 1990; 98:230.

Lindsay KL, Reynolds TB, Hoefs JC, San Marco ME. Specialty conference: Ascites. West J Med 1981; 134:414–423.

GASEOUSNESS

J. Edward Berk, M.D., D.Sc.

12

Symptoms conventionally considered to be related to excessive gastrointestinal gas are commonplace and a frequent cause for medical consultation. Yet, so-called gaseousness and its clinical expressions have from time immemorial been taken lightly and referred to jocularly. Reflecting this are certain incidents that dot the historical background of gastrointestinal gas, humorously alluded to by Levitt:[1] the selection by Hippocrates of "The Winds" as the title for his treatise on gastrointestinal gas and the disorders attributed to it; the formulation of a law by the fastidious Romans of the Caesars forbidding the expulsion of gas in public places; and the legendary Le Petomane whose amazing ability to inhale and exhale gas through his anus allowed him to perform feats such as "playing" popular tunes of the day. To these may be added the acceptance of the passage of "gas" as a form of parlor entertainment in Elizabethan England; the practice in some collegiate fraternal circles, perhaps still observed, of holding a lit match close to the anus of an initiate as gas is expelled to see if the gas will burn with a blue flame; and the repartée attributed to President William Howard Taft following his introduction at a public gathering.

The portly President had just been tastelessly presented by the noted orator, Chauncey Depew, as "the pregnant President Taft." When he rose to speak, President Taft commented that he and his wife had indeed discussed the situation to which Mr. Depew had alluded. They had decided that should it be a girl, she would be named after Mrs. Taft; should it be a boy, he would be named after the President. However, the President added, if he expelled what he thought it was, he would name it Chauncey De*pew!*

It is small wonder, then, that gaseousness tends to be treated cavalierly and is not accorded the degree of analytic concern that other gastrointestinal symptoms receive. It also is not surprising that the clinical perception of the underlying mechanisms responsible for the symptoms that may attend this disorder are all too often given inadequate consideration.

The intent of this chapter is to present a reasoned clinical analysis of this symptom complex. Such an evaluation cannot be made, however, without an appreciation of the nature and genesis of gastrointestinal gas. What follows, therefore, represents a summary of the currently established fundamentals.

Genesis and Composition of Gastrointestinal Gas

Volume of Gastrointestinal Gas in Normal Subjects

Gas normally is present in the gastrointestinal tract of adults. Measured in terms of the volume of gas washed out by argon introduced into the gut at about the level of the ligament of Treitz, Lasser and co-workers[2] found that the mean volume of gas present in the gut in a group of 10 normal adults was approximately 200 ml (199 ± 31 ml). These limited data additionally confirm that there is marked variation from person to person in the volume of intraluminal gas. Thus, assuming that the mean volume ± 2 standard deviations (SD) will encompass 95 percent of the normal population of adults, it may be concluded from the values obtained by Lasser and associates that the volume of intraluminal intestinal gas in the vast majority of normal persons varies from 137 to 261 ml.

> "*Gaseousness tends to be viewed and treated cavalierly.*"

Using as a parameter the less sophisticated technique of measuring the volume of gas collected in a bag attached to a rectal tube, it has been estimated that 400 to 1,200 ml of gas are expelled daily.[3] Aside from technical factors, the amount of gas recovered in this manner is influenced by the composition of the diet consumed and the bacterial flora of the gut.

Normal Expulsive Events

Gas within the gastrointestinal tract normally is reduced principally by absorption into the blood, by expulsion through the mouth (belching), and by expulsion through the anus (passage of flatus).

With respect to belching, no data are available on the frequency with which this occurs in healthy, normal adults. Notably lacking, therefore, is a quantitative standard for what is abnormal.

Information regarding how many times each day healthy persons expel flatus is extremely limited, but some data are available. In a study by Levitt and colleagues, seven normal young adults kept careful records of their daily

---

"Gas normally is present in the gastrointestinal tract of adults."

---

expulsions of flatus for a period of 1 week.[4] The mean daily number of passages of gas in this group was 13.6 ± 5.6 (1 SD). Adding 2 SD (11.2) to the mean volume of 13.6, which statistically should encompass 95 percent of the population, would establish the upper limit of normal as 25 passages a day.

Composition of Gastrointestinal Gas

Approximately 99 percent of the gas present in the gastrointestinal tract of normal adults is composed of five gases: nitrogen (N), oxygen (O), carbon dioxide (CO_2), hydrogen (H), and methane (CH_4) (Table 12–1). All these gases are odorless. The unpleasant odor that may be detected in flatus probably is imparted by (1) other gases that are present in trace amounts in the gut, and (2) hydrogen sulfide and mercaptans metabolized from sulfur-containing substances present in certain foods.

Sources of Gastrointestinal Gas

Of the five principal gases found in the gastrointestinal tract, only *nitrogen* and *oxygen* are present in material degree in atmospheric air. These are the gases, therefore, that enter the digestive tract when air is swallowed. The other three gases arise primarily within the gut (Fig. 12–1).

TABLE 12–1. Composition of Gastrointestinal Gas

Gas	Stomach (%)	Intestine (%)	Flatus (%)
Nitrogen (N_2)	79	23–80	11–92
Oxygen (O_2)	17	0.1–2.3	0–11
Carbon dioxide (CO_2)	4	5.1–29	3–54
Hydrogen (H_2)	–	0.06–47	0–69
Methane (CH_4)	–	0–26	0–56

Data from Roth JLA. Gaseousness. In: Berk JE, Haubrich WS, Kalser MH, Roth JLA, Schaffner F, eds. Bockus Gastroenterology. 4th ed. Philadelphia: WB Saunders, 1985:144.

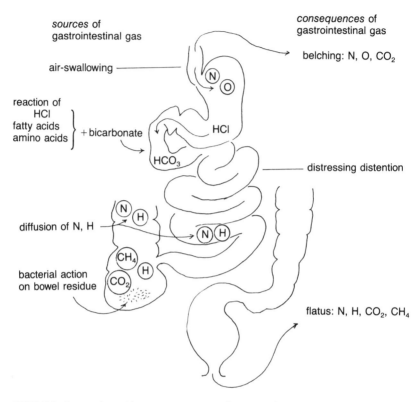

sources of
gastrointestinal gas

air-swallowing

reaction of
HCl
fatty acids } + bicarbonate
amino acids

HCl

HCO₃

consequences of
gastrointestinal gas

belching: N, O, CO₂

distressing distention

diffusion of N, H

bacterial action
on bowel residue

flatus: N, H, CO₂, CH₄

FIGURE 12-1.   Sources and potential symptomatic consequences of gastrointestinal gas.

Carbon dioxide is generated in surprisingly large amounts in the duodenum by the interaction between hydrochloric acid in gastric juice entering the duodenum and bicarbonate present in the duodenal contents. Carbon dioxide also is formed as a product of the reaction of bicarbonate with organic acids that result from fermentation in the gut.

"*F*ive gases account for 99 percent of the gas normally present in the gut of adults."

Hydrogen arises from bacterial metabolic processes that are active in the colon. The formation of hydrogen is most pronounced when fermentable carbohydrates in the diet are inadequately absorbed in the small bowel and become exposed to bacterial action on entering the colon.

Methane is formed in human beings solely from the metabolic activity of specific colonic bacteria. Bacterial organisms with the propensity to produce methane seem capable of acting not only on unabsorbed carbohydrates but also on substrates endogenous to the gut. It is notable that methane-forming bacteria are present in the colon in only one-third of the population; moreover, their existence has a familial linkage.

Clinical Features of Gaseousness

The complaints described by patients with gaseousness generally consist of (1) belching; (2) bloating, fullness, and abdominal discomfort; and (3) excessive expulsion of flatus (Fig. 12–2). Only infrequently does a given patient complain of any two of these symptoms; and rarely of all three. For this reason, and because they arise from different mechanisms, the three major clinical expressions of gaseousness are analyzed separately.

Belching

Illustrative Case

The patient, an obese 44-year-old mother of two children, decided to consult a physician after years of frequent, almost incessant belching, "My stomach," she said, "is loaded with gas, and I always feel blown up." Avoidance of gas-forming

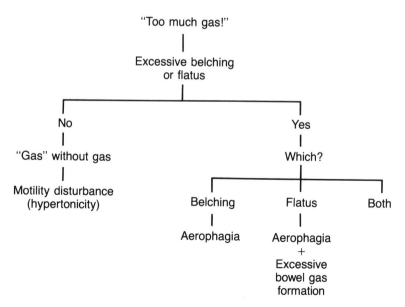

FIGURE 12–2. "Gaseousness" complex.

foods, as well as the use of a variety of drugs supposed to combat or reduce gas, had been to no avail.

Throughout the interview, she gave vent to loud, rumbling belches, after each of which she would clasp her hand to her mouth and state apologetically "I'm sorry."

Aside from obesity and the presence of an incisional scar in the right upper abdomen marking an elective cholecystectomy for gallstones 6 years earlier, physical examination was unremarkable.

Comment. This patient is a classic example of a natural phenomenon gone awry. Belching is a normal event experienced by everyone at some time, especially after a large meal or after a meal eaten rapidly. Belching is abnormal, however, when its frequency extends beyond that in the average healthy person. As already noted, "normal" frequency cannot be defined in quantitative terms, based on our present state of knowledge. The clinician is required, therefore, to determine empirically whether the frequency of belching in a given patient is exorbitant and clearly beyond normal bounds.

A telltale characteristic of the individual moved to seek medical advice for chronic, repetitive belching is the unabashed, public display of the act. A mild apology is often proffered when belching occurs in the company of others, but uninhibited repetition of belching is the rule.

In the patient with incessant, repetitive belching, *aerophagia* (air-swallowing) almost invariably plays a vital role. Close observation of the patient with repetitious belching will disclose that each eructation is preceded, often surreptitiously, by the aspiration and swallowing of air. This can be seen very clearly if the patient is capable of belching at will and obliges by doing so.

If the patient is observed fluoroscopically during the act of belching, air-swallowing is obvious preceding each belch. Roentgenograms of the upper abdomen taken before and after repeated belching will disclose that the *magenblase* (stomach bubble) normally present in the upper part of the stomach remains unchanged or is increased. This indicates that much of the swallowed air is promptly regurgitated from the esophagus with only variable portions reaching the stomach. Triphasic fluoroscopy, an assemblage of techniques for appraising swallowing function, may even more dramatically give objective evidence of air-swallowing and the degree to which the air is promptly eructated from the esophagus.

For purposes of understanding, it is very important that the patient is familiarized with the interrelationship of air-swallowing and chronic, habitual belching. This may be demonstrated fairly convincingly by several maneuvers:

1. Have the patient stand before a mirror and watch herself or himself closely while going through the act of belching. Call attention particularly to the aspiration of air that immediately precedes the belch.
2. Ask the patient to belch while biting hard on a bottle cork, or less effective, the eraser of a pencil. In most instances, belching will not be

possible because the biting prevents simultaneous air-swallowing. Some habitual belchers, however, manage to suck in some air despite the impediment.

3. Grasp the patient's trachea firmly at about the level of the thyroid cartilage and then ask the patient to belch. The fixation of the trachea interferes with swallowing and makes belching impossible.

"Belching and expulsion of flatus are normal events."

Although the purposeful but commonly unappreciated aspiration of atmospheric air is the prominent feature in patients with so-called malignant belching,[1,5] air may be aspirated and swallowed in other ways:[6]

1. When liquids or solid foods are bolted or eaten rapidly.
2. In the course of talking, especially talking while eating.
3. While sucking on objects such as a cigarette, cigar, or pipe.
4. While sipping liquids, especially from a saucer or other flat container.
5. While drinking liquids through a straw.
6. While chewing gum or sucking on candy.
7. Incidental to frequent swallowing induced by:
   a. Uncomfortable dentures.
   b. Dryness of the mouth for whatever reason, including mouth breathing during sleep.
   c. Postnasal drip.
   d. Asthmatic episodes with forcefully labored inspiration.
   e. Heartburn, which the patient may attempt to relieve by swallowing saliva.
   f. Stressful states—both physical, such as angina pectoris, and emotional, such as situations marked by acute surprise or embarrassment.
8. Because of impaired swallowing, as that due to bulbar or pseudobulbar palsy.

Gas entering the stomach as a consequence of one or more of the foregoing actions may be sufficient to enlarge the gastric gas bubble and distend the wall of the stomach. Should the individual elect to lie down following any of these actions, the air in the stomach will be unable to be expelled by eructation because intragastric fluid displaces it from the gastroesophageal opening. As a consequence, the air tends to move into the duodenum and is rapidly propelled through the gut. Indicative of the sometimes incredible rapidity of passage of swallowed air through the gut is the copious expulsion of flatus that may occur in the course of peroral endoscopy when the stomach has been insufflated with air. Depending on the volume advancing into the gut, segments of the bowel may become distended, producing a sense of fullness and abdominal discomfort.

"Incessant, repetitive belching is almost invariably associated with aerophagia."

Some of the swallowed air may extend as far as the left colon. Because the splenic flexure is the highest segment of the colon, and because gas tends to rise, the splenic flexure may become distended by gas. The same situation obtains in the lower-lying hepatic flexure. Gas is even more likely to accumulate in these flexures if, in addition to copious amounts of swallowed air, large volumes of gas are formed in the colon from bacterial metabolism of food residues (see the section, "Excessive Expulsion of Flatus"). Segmental colonic distention ensuing from the entrapped gas may induce symptom complexes named after the flexure affected (e.g., splenic flexure syndrome, hepatic flexure syndrome) (Fig. 12–3). The symptomatic expressions of these syndromes include bloating, fullness, and left or right upper abdominal discomfort depending on which flexure is distended (See Chapter 2, "Abdominal Pain").

It was mentioned earlier that an appreciable amount of air may find its way into the stomach in patients with heartburn who also hypersalivate and, because of this, swallow frequently. Conversely, heartburn may be provoked by

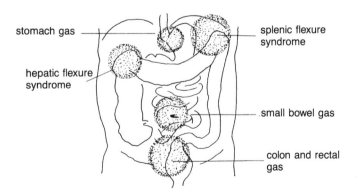

stomach gas

splenic flexure syndrome

hepatic flexure syndrome

small bowel gas

colon and rectal gas

FIGURE 12–3. Areas where collections of gas may produce discomfort.

the act of belching. This is particularly true in those with coexistent hiatus hernia and reduced lower esophageal sphincter pressure.

A special word of caution is in order with respect to air-swallowing in stressful states. Of particular concern in this regard is the patient with coronary artery disease who experiences angina pectoris or who may actually have an episode of myocardial infarction. The chest pain in such patients seems to trigger aerophagia. The clinical threat that this association imposes is the possibility that the discomfort may be attributed to gas distention and the basic lesion may be overlooked.

Bearing these several considerations in mind, the alert clinician will consider the possibility of some other coexistent disorder in a belcher whose belching is of recent onset, or in one who also experiences chest or abdominal pain. Appropriate studies aimed at identifying or excluding a concomitant abnormality should be undertaken in such circumstances.

Aside from air swallowed in the course of eating, air may enter the stomach in ingested food, both natural and prepared. Carbonated beverages and whipped foods, such as soufflés, are obvious examples of foodstuffs that are rich in air content. A raw apple would hardly be suspected of being a gas contributor, yet this fruit is considered to contain 20 percent gas by volume. Ingestion of such gas-containing foods in large amounts, particularly when ingested rapidly or when chewed and swallowed while talking, may likewise induce eructation to allow escape of air from the stomach.

Still another way that gas may find its way into the gastrointestinal tract is by diffusion from the blood. This occurs when the osmotic pressure of the gas in the blood is greater than that of the same gas in the lumen of the gut.

Studies to Consider. Objective evidence that the belching is associated with air-swallowing may be obtained by fluoroscopic examination during the act of swallowing a radiopaque liquid substance such as barium. The obvious presence in the barium column of air bubbles of variable size and number is clear evidence of aerophagia. If the patient should belch during this procedure, it may be observed that much of the swallowed air is expelled with the belch and fails to reach the stomach.

Comparison of films of the upper abdominal–lower chest region, taken before the ingestion of barium and again on completion of the contrast-meal study, may provide further support for simple air-swallowing as the principal cause of repetitive belching. If belching occurring during the examination represented expulsion of gas from within the stomach, the magenblase should diminish in size. Failure for this to occur or if there is an actual increase in its size constitutes evidence that the gas expelled in the act of belching was not of gastric origin.

Chemical analysis of gas aspirated from the stomach of a patient with frequent, repeated belching will disclose that the component gases are principally nitrogen and oxygen. Since these gases are the only intestinal gases present in atmospheric air, as noted earlier, their dominance in the stomach confirms the presence of aerophagia.

Although these approaches serve to corroborate air swallowing, they are not essential in the clinical assessment and management of the patient with no complaint other than habitual, repetitive belching. This is not the case, however, when the malignant belching is associated with other symptoms, notably pain of any type, regurgitation, or heartburn.

When such symptoms are described in addition to chronic belching, appropriate examinations should be made to ascertain their basis. Depending on the nature of the associated symptoms, the following studies may be advisable:

1. Plain film radiography of the abdomen to determine if there is gas accumulation in the gut, especially the splenic or hepatic flexure.
2. Barium esophagography to assess swallowing function and to determine if there is esophagogastric reflux or a hiatus hernia.
3. Esophagogastroduodenoscopy to determine if there are signs of esophagitis, erosive gastritis, or peptic ulcer disease.

If pain is a complaint, and especially if it is situated in the lower sternal region, angiographic and related studies to assess coronary circulation and myocardial function may well be in order.

"Gas accumulation in the colonic flexures and elsewhere in the gastrointestinal tract may cause distressing symptoms."

Sometimes an aerophagic person will complain of upper abdominal discomfort and fullness suggestive of gaseous distention in one of the areas where gastrointestinal gas tends to accumulate (see Fig. 12–3), but a plain film of the abdomen discloses little or no gas entrapment in these locales. The situation in such instances may be clarified by maneuvers aimed at reproducing the symptoms. As an example, air may be insufflated into the colon through a rectal tube in amounts sufficient to distend the splenic and the hepatic flexures. Reproduction of the discomfort that has been distressing the patient lends support to the clinical suspicion of gas-induced splenic or hepatic flexure syndrome.

Examinations Performed. Radiographic examination of the upper gastrointestinal tract was made before and after spontaneous belching and after the ingestion of barium. It was noted that (1) a great deal of air was swallowed,

(2) the gas bubble in the stomach increased slightly after repeated episodes of belching, and (3) the stomach and duodenum appeared morphologically normal.

Consideration was given to complementary esophagogastroduodenoscopy on the strength of the possibility that there might be some lesion masked by the frequent belching. However, because of the long duration of the belching, the unimpaired nutrition, the patient's general good health, and the lack of roentgenologically evident disease in the upper gastrointestinal tract, no other special studies were carried out.

Management. The role of air-swallowing in chronic, persistent, repetitive belching was carefully described and demonstrated to the patient. Emphasis was placed on the habitual nature of the belching and the need to repress the urge to belch. The patient was advised to eat slowly, to chew her food well, and to avoid talking at length while eating. Carbonated beverages, gum chewing, smoking, and sucking on candies and similar articles were all proscribed.

No medications were considered necessary. Gas absorbers, such as charcoal, and agents that act to coalesce small bubbles of gas, such as simethicone (Mylicon), were considered but were concluded to be of dubious value in instances of repetitive air-swallowing. Antacids were also considered to reduce the amount of acid entering the duodenum and hence lead to smaller amounts of CO_2 being formed. They were not prescribed, however, because it was surmised that the contribution would be of minimal clinical value at best in a patient whose major complaint was repetitive belching.

Prognosis. The prognosis was guarded. It was thought likely that belching would be reduced if the program outlined was followed, but that the condition would not be abolished.

Bloating, Fullness, and Abdominal Discomfort

☐ *Illustrative Case*

A 36-year-old woman was referred because of bloating and abdominal pain dating back to her high-school days. Although her general health was maintained throughout this time, she scarcely had a single day without abdominal distress. Because of this, she had consulted numerous physicians and undergone repeated examinations and special studies. Among the latter were barium-meal examination of the upper gastrointestinal tract, barium enema, oral cholecystography, proctosigmoidoscopy, ultrasonography, and computed tomographic examination of the abdomen. None of these examinations disclosed an abnormality.

The patient had been advised to avoid gas-forming foods and had been given a variety of medications. While some of the drugs were helpful for a while, the distress inevitably recurred.

The patient stated, "Doctor, I'm a gas former. Everything I eat turns to gas—and it's killing me." Her symptoms consisted principally of a bloated feeling and abdominal discomfort, most pronounced shortly after eating. The abdominal discomfort was generally mild to moderate in severity, was variably located, and occurred almost daily but without a regular pattern of time of appearance.

The physical examination was unremarkable.

Comment. The symptom complex of bloating, fullness, and abdominal discomfort are popularly classified under the rubric "gaseousness." The same subjective complaints, however, are encountered in a number of digestive tract disorders, both organic and so-called functional. This complex, therefore, must be regarded as nonspecific. Nevertheless, there is a subset of patients who complain principally of these sensations and who are convinced that the symptoms result from excessive intestinal gas. Despite this conviction, it is notable that many adamantly deny belching or expelling flatus to excess, and many obtain no relief from expulsion of gas.

The patient whose case history is described here is representative of this group. The seeming plausibility of a cause-and-effect relationship between the symptoms that she so vividly expressed and gas accumulation in the gut, coupled with the lack of a reliable means of measuring the quantity of intestinal gas, have encouraged general acceptance of the hypothesis that this symptom complex is gas-related.

The primary challenge to the discerning clinician when dealing with a patient with such complaints is to determine whether the symptoms are indeed related to or arising from increased intestinal gas. To meet this challenge, it is helpful to bear in mind certain pertinent data that bear importantly on this subject.

> *"Bloating, fullness, and abdominal discomfort may arise from factors other than excessive intestinal gas."*

Although much remains to be learned, studies made by Lasser and colleagues in 1975 provide no support for the long-cherished notion that the sensations of bloating, fullness, and abdominal discomfort are related to abnormal accumulations of gas in the gut.[2] To obtain objective information, these investigators employed an intestinal gas washout technique that featured infusion into the upper jejunum of a mixture of 95 percent argon and 5 percent sulfur hexafluoride. All gas washed out of the rectum was collected, measured, and analyzed. The stomach was also constantly aspirated during the infusion, and the amount of argon infusate that refluxed into the stomach was calculated from the volumes of sulfur hexafluoride recovered.

In this study, one group consisted of 12 patients with chronic complaints attributed to excessive intestinal gas. The volume of gas in their intestinal tracts proved to be no different than that measured similarly in another group made up of 10 control subjects. In contrast to the controls, however, the patients presumed to have excess gas experienced abdominal pain after infusion of volumes of gas that gave the subjects in the control group no distress. In addition, in the suspect gaseous patients, more of the gas tended to reflux into the stomach, and the intestinal transit time of the infused gas was longer than that in the control group.

These observations clearly indicate that—contrary to conventional wisdom, the patient's conviction, and the attending physician's suspicion—chronic bloating, fullness, and abdominal discomfort in these patients did not originate in excessive intestinal gas. Rather, the responsible mechanisms appeared to involve disordered intestinal motility and a heightened pain response to intestinal distention.

It follows from the findings of Lasser and co-workers that the symptom complex of chronic persistent bloating, fullness, and abdominal discomfort should be reclassified. Instead of categorizing this complex as a form of gaseousness, as has long been the case, it would perhaps be better classified as a gastrointestinal motility disorder. Before making this taxonomic switch, however, certain caveats must be sounded.

Neither previous observations, such as those of Oppenheimer,[7] who was unable to detect evidence of increased intestinal gas in plain films of the abdomen of patients complaining of "gas pains," nor the studies of Lasser and associates showing normal intestinal gas volumes in patients with the chronic "gas syndrome," totally exclude intestinal gas as a contributor to the abdominal disquietude that torments these unfortunate patients. There is no absolute correlation between the volume of gas seen on a plain film of the abdomen at a given time and the occurrence of symptoms; large amounts of gas may be evident without any subjective symptoms, and vice versa. The total volume of gas may be within normal limits, yet an isolated loop or loops of bowel may be temporarily overdistended with gas. Moreover, the fact that a patient with the symptom complex of chronic bloating, fullness, and abdominal discomfort experiences discomfort when gas is introduced into his or her gut in comparatively small volumes suggests that gas per se may trigger symptoms even though the total quantity of gas is not greater than in asymptomatic subjects.

Further attesting to the potential of gas within the lumen of the bowel independently to invoke abdominal discomfort are the feelings of bloating and fullness that may be associated simply with pronounced aerophagia (see the previous section, "Belching"). It is all the more likely, then, that gas itself may be a factor should the chronic "excess gas former" also be an air-swallower.

A heavy milk-drinker who is lactase-deficient may form enormous amounts of gas.[4] Some of the gas may reflux into the small bowel, distend one or more segments, and, as a consequence, aggravate the discomfort caused by the large volume of gas formed by bacterial action on undigested lactose reaching the colon.

Patients with extensive enteritis may not only be lactase-deficient because of widespread mucosal damage, which diminishes further what lactase activity had previously been present, but may also have small intestinal bacterial overgrowth. The action of these bacteria on the undigested lactose in the lumen of the small bowel may result in gas accumulation sufficient to distend a loop of small bowel and to produce an uncomfortable feeling of distention.

Patients with intestinal pseudo-obstruction, a disorder in which intestinal motility is markedly abnormal, may have marked gaseous distention and may commonly experience symptoms that include bloating, fullness, and abdominal discomfort.

Despite these and other situations in which it is conceivable that gaseous distention may underlie symptoms of bloating, fullness, and abdominal discomfort, it seems wiser to focus primary attention on intestinal motility derangement in patients who chronically suffer such complaints but are otherwise in good health. To do so is in keeping with current knowledge and makes possible more precise and reasoned classification. Furthermore, therapy can be centered on measures that may beneficially affect motor function of the gut rather than on medications and dietary maneuvers designed to reduce, absorb, or physically modify intestinal gas. Whether such a change in therapeutic focus will yield better clinical results remains to be seen. Certainly, clinical experience has made it clear that anti-gas measures are not attended by longlasting benefit in these unfortunate individuals.

"Intestinal motility derangement appears principally responsible for 'gaseous' symptoms of bloating, fullness, and abdominal discomfort."

Studies to Consider. As noted earlier, the patient whose encapsulated case history introduced this section is typical of the subset of patients with chronic complaints of bloating, fullness, and abdominal discomfort popularly attributed to gaseous distention of the gut. The very chronicity of her distress, her relatively young age, the lack of other arresting symptoms—all decry the need for intensive investigation. If the patient were to reject the notion of intestinal dysmotility and cling tenaciously to her conviction that the problem was essentially excessive intestinal gas, it might be helpful to obtain a plain film of the abdomen while she was experiencing distress. Failure of this examination to disclose an increased volume of intestinal gas would provide evidence against excessive gas, even though it would not truly eliminate gas as a contributing factor.

If the need were even more desperate, or if the attending physician were not fully satisfied, a small tube could be inserted into the upper small intestine and a quantity of room air instilled. Prompt reproduction of the discomfort spontaneously experienced, especially after instillation of only a small amount of air, should provide convincing evidence of at least overresponsiveness of the gut to gaseous distention.

More complex diagnostic maneuvers, such as argon washout of the gut to prove that total intestinal gas content is not abnormally increased, are unnecessary even if such sophisticated experimental studies could be accomplished.

In older patients, especially those whose symptoms are of fairly recent origin, and in patients of any age who present additional symptoms such as weight loss, vomiting, diarrhea, or gross or occult bleeding, standard examinations of the gastrointestinal tract are required to exclude organic disease. Among the studies to consider would be imaging techniques (e.g., conventional radiography, abdominal sonography, and computed tomography) and endoscopy.

Management.   The concept of disturbed intestinal motility with lowered threshold of pain perception by the gut was diligently explained to the patient. She was assured that the nature of the symptoms, their long duration, her generally good health, and the uniformly negative findings of the numerous diagnostic procedures that had already been carried out indicated that there was no organic disorder.

"The so-called gas syndrome of bloating, fullness, and abdominal discomfort presents a therapeutic challenge."

Even though the patient was not forming gas in excessive quantity, the irritability of the gut and its tendency to overrespond to even small amounts of gas made it reasonable to try to diminish the volume of gas in the intestines. Therefore, the patient was counseled about air-swallowing (see the previous section, "Belching"), advised to eliminate such legumes as beans and other notorious gas-forming foods from her diet, and either to avoid milk and milk-containing products or to supplement their ingestion with a lactase preparation taken beforehand (see the following section, "Excessive Expulsion of Flatus"). She was additionally advised to reduce fiber intake, particularly bran.

Metoclopramide (Reglan), which the patient had taken previously with benefit for a short time, was again prescribed. When other, probably more effective prokinetic drugs (e.g., domperidone, cisapride) are ultimately approved for clinical use in the United States, one of these will likely be substituted.

Prognosis.   The patient has not been seen since the foregoing program was recommended. Based on widely shared clinical experience, it is uncertain whether the regimen outlined will be beneficial. Unfortunately, clinical improvement, if it does occur, most likely will not be longlasting. In all probability, repeated reassurance and the ultimate use of more effective prokinetic drugs will be required.

Excessive Expulsion of Flatus

Genesis and Composition of Flatus

The genesis of intestinal gas and its composition are summarized above. Some of the features noted in this summary have particular bearing on the problem of flatulence and therefore are reiterated for emphasis.

Gas expulsion from the rectum is, of course, a normal event. The amount of hard data on this natural phenomenon, however, are incredibly sparse. Based on observations made by Levitt and colleagues in a group of seven young men,[4] up to 25 expulsions of gas may occur normally each day.

The five gases that account for 99 percent of the intestinal gas normally present in the gut (see Table 12–1) also may be found in expelled flatus in normal persons. Oxygen is found only in minimal amounts because of its utilization by the mucosal cells, or the bacteria in the gut, or both. Nitrogen ordinarily accounts for a large proportion, and methane is found only in the one-third of the population with the capacity to form it. In patients with a greater than normal frequency of gaseous discharges, hydrogen and carbon dioxide, along with methane, are the dominant gases present.

The oxygen detectable in the flatus of patients with excessive gas passages probably originates in swallowed air. The nitrogen present also may have originated in swallowed air, but presently available information and study methods provide no reliable means of separating or distinguishing how much luminal nitrogen is attributable to swallowed air, and how much to diffusion from the blood. Hydrogen and methane arise from within the lumen of the colon as the result of bacterial action on carbohydrate food residues that escape digestion in the small bowel. Carbon dioxide is also generated intraluminally but at two different sites and through two different mechanisms (as described previously). In the upper small intestine, it is released in the process of neutralization of hydrochloric acid or fatty acids by bicarbonate; in the lower bowel, it is the result of bacterial action, especially on fermentable carbohydrate residues. Carbon dioxide formed in the upper gut is rapidly absorbed so that little or none reaches the colon. The large amount of carbon dioxide in flatus, therefore, most likely is the product of bacterial metabolism in the lower bowel.

Without any explosive sound arising in the course of passage of gas from the anus, or any offensive odor, gas may be expelled without other people in close proximity being aware of the act. Not too well appreciated is the fact that the major intestinal gases have no odor detectable by the human olfactory system. When flatus is malodorous, as is often the case, the offensive odor is attributable to the formation of other gases that ordinarily are present in only trace amounts. An unpleasant odor may also be imparted to the flatus by the formation of hydrogen sulfide and mercaptans from sulfur-containing substances found in certain foods.

Pathophysiology of Excessive Flatus

The foregoing basic information regarding flatus is essential to the management of the patient complaining of excessive expulsion of gas. When the normal process of rectal gaseous discharge becomes symptomatic because of "excessive" frequency, primary attention should center on aerophagia, food intake, digestion and absorption, and bacterial activity in the gut.

Aerophagia.   The symptom of inordinate belching was considered previously in the section, "Belching." In the discussion of this troubling symptom, considerable emphasis was placed on air-swallowing, or aerophagia. Many patients who expel flatus excessively also swallow considerable amounts of air

"Excessive expulsion of flatus may have several causes."

in the course of their daily activities. Some aggravate this by being habitual belchers. To what extent air that is swallowed, or that enters with food, contributes to excessive flatus is uncertain and at present cannot be assessed accurately. Although aerophagia probably is not the dominant factor responsible for exaggerated expulsions of flutus, it seems reasonable to assign it at least a contributory role,[6] even in patients with small gut dysrhythmia (see the previous section, "Bloating, Fullness, and Abdominal Discomfort").

The occurrence of such phenomena as the splenic flexure syndrome in aerophagic patients (see the section, "Belching," and Chapter 2, "Abdominal Pain") suggests that a substantial amount of swallowed air may traverse the gut for such a distance, especially when air-swallowing is of marked degree. Whatever air does get that far, when added to the large volumes of gas that may form within the colon in some persons (see below), provides a combination that may lead to gas entrapment in the high-lying splenic flexure and to subsequent distention of this segment of the colon.

Gas Formation Within the Gut.   Chemical interaction, in the first part of the duodenum, between hydrochloric acid discharged by the stomach and the bicarbonate in the duodenal lumen produces an amazing quantity of carbon dioxide. Levitt has pointed out that 1 mEq of hydrochloric acid reacting with 1 mEq of bicarbonate releases about 22.8 ml of carbon dioxide.[1] Neutralization by bicarbonate of an estimated average postcibal gastric secretion of 30 mEq of hydrochloric acid per hour would release 700 ml of carbon dioxide per hour.

Reaction between duodenal bicarbonate and the fatty acids released when triglycerides are acted on in the duodenum by pancreatic lipase also produces carbon dioxide. Levitt noted that neutralization by duodenal bicarbonate of 100 mEq of fatty acids (an amount that could be released after a large meal) would yield 2,000 ml of carbon dioxide.[1]

The rich bacterial flora within the colon act on food residues that escape complete digestion and absorption in the higher reaches of the gut. Fermentation reactions that they induce, especially on carbohydrate residues, result in metabolic products such as hydrogen, carbon dioxide, and methane. Some hydrogen may be derived directly from hydrogen-forming bacteria, and some carbon dioxide may result indirectly from the reaction between bicarbonate and organic acids found in the process of bacterial fermentation. Methane is formed only in colons that harbor the specific microbes capable of metabolizing this gas.

Diffusion from the Blood.   Bowel gases pass freely in either direction between the lumen of the gut and the blood, the direction depending on the partial pressure gradient for each gas. The volume of a gas at a given time in a given segment of the gut may be regarded as the resultant of the partial pressure gradients and the equilibrium attained between the gas in the gut and that in the blood. The quantities of the several gases in flatus are influenced by the same operative factors.

Two aspects of the diffusion and equilibration phenomena of intestinal gas have practical diagnostic application. Inasmuch as hydrogen is derived from metabolic actions of bacteria on fermentable substrates, or perhaps in part by direct secretion by some bacteria, the site of its formation in normal persons may be considered to be essentially confined to the colon. The sudden addition of hydrogen dilutes the other gases in the lumen of the colon and they equilibrate rapidly with the blood. As a consequence, the partial pressure of the nitrogen in the colonic lumen falls, and nitrogen diffuses from the blood to establish equilibrium. When the other gases are increased, the balancing process results in an increase of nitrogen as well. Hence the gas passed from the rectum will contain large volumes of nitrogen along with large quantities of carbon dioxide, hydrogen, and possibly methane. Accordingly, the presence of large amounts of nitrogen in the flatus of a patient with excessive expulsion of rectal gas cannot in itself be considered evidence that the excessive flatus is due primarily to air-swallowing. Such a conclusion might be warranted if a sample of flatus contained mainly nitrogen. In contrast, when carbon dioxide, hydrogen, and perhaps methane are the principal gases, bacterial action on a fermentable substrate probably is the source of the gas. The concomitant large volume of nitrogen in the flatus in this circumstance probably reflects the diffusion adjustment just described. It is not possible, however, absolutely to exclude swallowed air as the source of some of the nitrogen.

The second diagnostically helpful application that stems from the diffusion characteristics of intestinal gas is the use of breath hydrogen excretion to measure hydrogen production in the gut. Because the concentration of hydrogen in the lumen of the colon, where it is generated, is always higher than in the blood, hydrogen is regularly in process of diffusion into the blood flowing through the colon. In the blood it is carried to the lungs, where it is removed and excreted in expired air. Measurement of the amount of hydrogen excreted in the breath, therefore, provides a useful means of assaying hydrogen production in the colon.

Nature of Food Consumed.   Gas may enter the stomach not only from the swallowing of atmospheric air but also in foods that are consumed. Prominent among such air-containing foods are whipped preparations, such as soufflés, and carbonated beverages. Solid foods may contain air in surprising amounts. Thus, for example, as previously noted, apples are said to contain 20 percent air.[1]

"Not all foodstuffs are completely digested and absorbed."

Although digestion and absorption in the small bowel is of a high order, not all foodstuffs are completely digested, even in normal persons. Dietary flours are incompletely absorbed, except for rice and gluten-free wheat flour. Ordinary table sugar (sucrose) is not entirely absorbed. Some legumes, notably beans, contain oligosaccharides (raffinose and stachyose) that are not broken down because the normal gut lacks the requisite enzymes to metabolize them. It is common knowledge today that many healthy persons are unable to metabolize lactose because they lack the enzyme lactase.

Foodstuffs may fail to be assimilated in the small intestine because of disorders that reduce pancreatic exocrine secretion, denude or destroy the mucosa of the small intestine, obstruct lymphatic drainage, or in other ways impair digestion and absorption. In these situations, the undigested or unabsorbed food elements reach the colon, where they are metabolized by the colonic bacteria, with the production, among other products, of gases.

Studies to Consider. Just as one would inquire at length about the number and character of the stool passages in a patient with a complaint of diarrhea (see Chapter 8, "Diarrhea"), so should one inquire about the frequency and peculiarities of the gas expulsions in a patient complaining of flatulence.

First and foremost, it should be established in some objective manner that the rectal gaseous discharges of which the patient complains is truly related to an excessive volume of intestinal gas. The data sought should either confirm that the gaseous discharges represent a departure from normal or rule out underlying excessive gastrointestinal gas. The latter is important, in part, because gaseousness, like many other gastrointestinal symptoms, must be interpreted with full recognition of cultural attitudes and individual personalities. For example, a prim matron might be alarmed as well as embarrassed by a solitary uncontrollable and publicly occurring expulsion of gas. In contrast, in certain cultural and racial groups gas expulsions, whether as a belch or as passage of flatus, are accepted as natural physiologic expressions and therefore are less apt to become complaints for which medical advice is solicited.

One way to gauge the complaint of excessive expulsion of gas is simply to ask the patient to record accurately the number of expulsions of gas occurring during a 24-hour period, assuming frequency to reflect volume and taking the outside upper limit to be 25 discharges per 24 hours, as previously noted. Knowing the actual daily frequency of rectal gaseous expulsions before instituting treatment also provides a baseline for evaluation of the effect of therapy. Notwithstanding these advantages, such information is rarely sought in clinical practice.

Should the number of gaseous passages recorded by the patient clearly exceed the noted upper limit of normal, the special examinations required to uncover the cause or causes depend on the clinical features in each patient. If the excessive flatus has been present for a long time and the patient's general health has not changed throughout this period, few studies are needed or are vital. In all cases, it would be wise to test for lactase deficiency by noting the effect of drinking cold milk after an overnight fast or, more specifically, by measuring the blood sugar response to a load of lactose (25 to 50 g) or the hydrogen level in expired air after oral administration of lactose. Also helpful would be a stool examination for undigested food remnants and for ova and parasites, especially *Giardia lamblia*. If the patient has identified certain foods, besides milk, that seem to aggravate the flatulence, these may be tested by a hydrogen breath test after their ingestion.

When the flatulence is fairly recent in appearance and is attended by other symptoms, such as abdominal discomfort, impaired appetite, weight loss, and change in bowel habit, radiographic and endoscopic studies of the gastrointestinal tract are warranted. Roentgenographic examination of the small intestine should include particular attention to transit time as well as to morphologic alterations in the small intestinal pattern.

In uncommon instances when excessive flatus is associated with frequent belching and pronounced aerophagia and it is uncertain whether air-swallowing or fermentation of undigested food remnants is responsible for the flatulence, or when dietary manipulation has not appreciably improved the complaint, the physician should consider gas analysis of the flatus. Such a sample may be easily collected by aspiration with a syringe attached to a rectal tube.[4] As noted earlier, if the sample is found to contain chiefly nitrogen, air-swallowing would be the likely cause for the excessive expulsions of flatus; if hydrogen and carbon dioxide (and perhaps methane) are the principal gases, it may be concluded that the condition results from bacterial action on maldigested or malabsorbed fermentable food residues.

A more elegant alternative, and one doubtless more appealing to both the patient and the physician, is a breath analysis for hydrogen. Heightened excretion of this gas in expired air is an index of the delivery to the colon of fermentable substrate and favors colonic bacterial fermentation as the basis for the flatulence.

Illustrative Case

A 35-year-old lawyer was referred because of frequent and uncontrollable passage of gas by rectum. He was uncertain just when this began but noted that his high-school classmates had made fun of him because of it. He was distressed and embarrassed by audible expulsions occurring while in discussion with a client or when he was appearing in court.

Passages of flatus had become more frequent during the previous 5 years. The patient could offer no reason to account for this, but on close questioning described himself as a "health nut." About the same time that the expulsions of flatus increased in frequency, he had adandoned meat and had begun to eat "health foods." His diet over this period was made up for the most part of cereals (including bran), nuts, whole-grain breads, salads, raw fruits, eggs, and milk and other dairy products. Aside from the large number of rectal passages of gas, the patient considered himself in good health. When pressed for more details regarding his dietary and living habits, the patient disclosed that he was fond of milk, consuming a quart or more daily. During the previous 5 years he had also become a devotee of wheat bran, taking no less than 4 heaping tablespoonfuls daily.

No abnormalities were noted on physical examination.

Examinations Performed. Because the patient complained only of excessive flatus for many years, because his general health was good, and because the physical examination was entirely negative, no special studies were made.

Management. An explanation was given to the patient of what was considered to be the basis for his excessive passage of flatus. Emphasis was placed on the need for him to modify his diet as directed.

Ingestion of ordinary milk and milk products, with the exception of yogurt, was proscribed. If there was clinical improvement, the patient was advised to try some milk pretreated with lactase or taken after the oral ingestion of lactase (commercially available as Lactaid and Lactrase).

A diet low in wheat, oats, and fiber was outlined, and rice and gluten-free flours were recommended as alternatives. The patient was counseled to avoid gas-forming foods, including legumes such as beans; vegetables such as cabbage, cauliflower, corn, cucumbers, Brussels sprouts, onions, turnips, soybeans, and radishes; and fruits such as melons, raw apples, and avocados.

> "*A*voidance of foods containing elements
> that are poorly absorbed is an important part
> of treatment."

It was further suggested that sodas and fruit juices containing fructose, and sugar-free foods containing sorbitol, be omitted. Inasmuch as both these substances are incompletely digested, their residues provide good substrates for bacterial metabolism and gas formation.

Although the patient denied belching excessively, he was informed about the adverse effect of aerophagia in his situation and urged to avoid air-swallowing by observing the precautionary measures detailed previously in the section, "Belching."

Because it might possibly help to diminish carbon dioxide formation in the duodenum by reducing the acid load, an antacid was prescribed to be taken after each meal. No other medications were ordered. Charcoal, whose absorbent effect is moot, was held in reserve for use if the response to the prescribed regimen was poor, or if the flatus became embarrassingly offensive in odor. Simethicone (Mylicon) was considered of no proven value, and administration of antibiotics to reduce the colonic flora was thought to have uncertain effects and, if effective, to be only of temporary value.

Prognosis. The patient was requested to continue to record the number of rectal gaseous expulsions experienced daily while on the program outlined. It was hoped that the regimen, if indeed carefully and closely observed, would improve the situation. Prognosis, however, was guarded and no conclusions could be drawn for some time.

References

1. Levitt M.D. Gastrointestinal gas and abdominal symptoms. Practical gastroenterology. Part 1. 1982; 7:6–12. Part 2. 1982; 8:6–14.
2. Lasser RB, Bond JH, Levitt MD. The role of intestinal gas in functional abdominal pain. N Engl J Med 1975; 293:524–526.
3. Berk JE, ed. Symposium on gastrointestinal gas. Ann NY Acad Sci, 1968.
4. Levitt MD, Lasser RB, Schwartz JS, Bond JH. Studies of a flatulent patient. N Engl J Med 1976; 295:260–262.
5. Levitt MD. Intestinal gas: what do we offer the patient? In: Barkin J, Rogers A, eds. Difficult decisions in digestive diseases. Chicago: Year Book, 1989:341–345.
6. Roth JLS. Gaseousness. In: Berk JE, Haubrich WS, Kalser MH, Roth JLA, Schaffner F, eds. Bockus Gastroenterology. 4th ed. Philadelphia: WB Saunders, 1985:142–166.
7. Oppenheimer A. Gas in the bowels: Observations and experiments in man. Surg Gynecol Obstet 1940; 70:105–114.

ANOREXIA

J. Edward Berk, M.D., D.Sc.

13

Of all the clinical expressions of disorders of the digestive system, probably none is more misconstrued than the symptom designated *anorexia*. This important and frequently encountered symptom cannot be intelligently interpreted or evaluated without a clear understanding of what it is and what it connotes. Accordingly, a glossary of terms is an appropriate introduction to its consideration (see also Fig. 13–1). In this regard, it should be noted that the focus in this chapter is on the symptom, anorexia. The eating disorder, anorexia nervosa, of which anorexia is a feature, is considered in Chapter 14, "Eating Disorders."

Glossary

Anorexia is derived from the Greek *an,* meaning "lack of," and *orexis,* meaning "appetite."[1] The terms from which it stems well define its meaning. Yet, the word is all too often misused in clinical practice and is not sharply distinguished from others that relate to diminished food intake.

It is more the rule than the exception to have a patient reply to the question "How is your appetite?" by a statement such as "I don't feel hungry." To accept a reply of this type unquestioningly courts misinterpretation and the danger of embarking on an investigational course that could prove unproductive as well as costly.

Hunger is a sensation completely different from appetite. It is a group or complex of sensations that come into play when there is physiologic need for

233

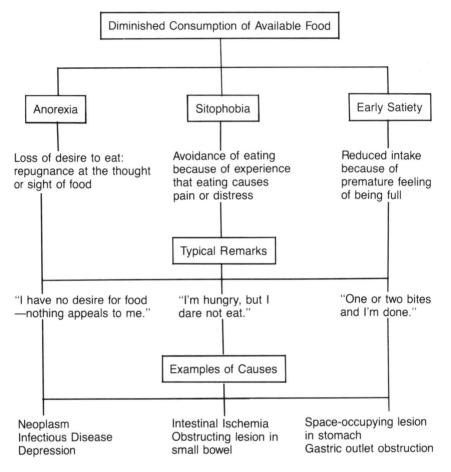

FIGURE 13-1. Diminished consumption of food and its causes.

"**H**unger *and* appetite *are not synonymous.*"

sustenance. Included among its manifestations are a feeling of emptiness, upper abdominal discomfort (classically identified as "hunger pangs"), weakness, irritability, sometimes headache, and occasionally sweating and trembling. The hunger state with all its manifold expressions abates and disappears promptly after the ingestion of food.

Anorexia signifies, not absence of hunger, but loss of *appetite.* This term and what it implies must be fully appreciated if anorexia is to be judged to truly exist. Appetite is derived from the Latin *appetitio,* meaning "craving"; this word, in turn, is a combination of the Latin prefix *ap* (toward) and the term *petitus* (desire).[1] It refers fundamentally to the desire for food but embraces within its connotation the element of anticipatory pleasure. The latter is born of the pleasant sensations associated with the partaking of agreeable foods and is further strengthened by the recollection of enticing aromas, pleasant taste sensations, and attractive settings.

Although frequently concurrent, hunger and appetite may exist independently. Thus, an individual may be hungry to the point of being desperate for food and yet have no appetite for the only food available if it is distasteful or proscribed by religious practice. An example would be pork set before a famished person whose religious faith has set a taboo on this food.

The converse situation would be an appetite-driven desire for dessert at the end of a meal, even though hunger was long since assuaged by the food already eaten. Consider in this regard the common experience of partaking in a long-anticipated banquet of multiple courses. The libations and hors d'oeuvres preceding the banquet proper probably satisfied any hunger that had been present—hunger likely aggravated by purposely omitting food earlier in the day to prepare for the sumptuous repast to be served. Nevertheless, appetite, abetted by enjoyment of everything already eaten, the ambience, the attractive service, and the nature of the occasion, encourages continued eating, even to the point of uncomfortable fullness. A belt may be unbuckled or a tight garment loosened to relieve the fullness, but eating is unchecked and continues merrily.

When questioning a possibly anorexic patient, one means of assuring that appetite has diminished or disappeared is to ask the patient to identify his or her favorite food. The patient is then asked "How would you like to have a well-done steak smothered in onions (or a schmaltz herring, or an enchilada, or whatever) right now?" If the answer is "You bet!" the patient does not have anorexia. But if the reply is "No thanks I couldn't eat it . . . It would just go to waste," then anorexia must be suspected.

"Appetite *is the* desire *for food; hunger is a complex of sensations that appear when there is physiological* need *for food."*

The next line of questioning should be directed at the reason for declining a food item previously cherished. If the reply to the question "Why couldn't you eat it—it's your favorite food, isn't it?" is to the effect that food in general, including the favorite food, is no longer appealing, it may be safely concluded that the patient does indeed have anorexia. But should the answer be "I feel too uncomfortable after I eat," then the nature of the postprandial discomfort must be clarified.

One way to approach this is to ask the patient to describe in his or her own words what is felt after eating, and how soon afterward the "uncomfortable" sensation appears. A volunteered statement such as "Almost as soon as I begin to eat, I get so much pain in my stomach I have to quit eating" would point to *sitophobia*. This condition is aptly defined by the words from which it originated: the Greek words *sitas,* meaning "food," and *phobein,* meaning "to fear."[1] Sitophobia is marked by refusal to eat for fear of pain that follows ingestion of food.

With suspicion of sitophobia in mind, I have found it useful to ask the following: "Suppose I could wave a magic wand and promise you that there would be absolutely no pain after you ate. Suppose I then set before you your favorite food, would you eat it?" An affirmative reply such as "Yes, I think so," and certainly an enthusiastic response such as "And how! Just bring it on," would confirm that there is no lack of desire for food, and that the problem rather is fear of the pain and discomfort precipitated by eating.

> **"S**itophobia *is refusal to eat for fear of pain after eating."*

If instead of describing pain or hurting, the patient pictures the "uncomfortable" feeling noted after eating in such words as "I used to be able to pack away a big meal without any problem. Now I get all filled up after a few bites or mouthfuls" then the impaired food consumption would appear ascribable to early satiety. The term *satiety,* derived from the Latin *satis,* meaning "enough,"[1] is related to the state attained when appetite has been fully gratified. *Early satiety* means that there is gratification of appetite by much less food than would ordinarily be expected to bring this about, or that was the case before.

Pathogenesis

Eating is so much a part of daily life that little thought is given to all the factors that are involved and that can influence when and what we eat. The intricate, many-faceted regulation of feeding has been succinctly summarized by Morley and co-workers as "an extremely complex process involving a variety of peripheral inputs including the hedonic qualities of food, neuronal and hormonal signals from the gastrointestinal tract, the physicochemical qualities of absorbed food, the state of glycogen stores in the liver, the status of the organism's fat stores, and possibly the activity of brown adipose tissue. In addition to these internal cues, external cues such as the availability and types of food, the psychological factors in higher animals and cultural factors (e.g., the need to eat only kosher food) in humans also play a role."[2]

Intimately involved in feeding control is the interaction between the "feeding center" in the lateral hypothalamus and the "satiety center" in the medial hypothalamic nuclei.[3] The anatomic location and functional contributions of these centers are predicated on observations of the effects of destructive lesions produced experimentally in these regions. Both centers affect feeding by their modulation of a host of reflex mechanisms involving receptors in various parts of the body, including the nervous system, the gastrointestinal system, and other, nongastrointestinal viscera.[4]

If one were to seek a simplistic view of the pathogenesis of anorexia set against the panoply of the regulation of feeding, one might be tempted to regard it as the product of heightened satiety sensation resulting from the interplay of many opposing stimuli and forces. Although attractive if for no reason other than its simplicity, this concept obscures the fact that anorexia is in essence a nonspecific symptom and that it may be associated with numerous bodily derangements, nondigestive as well as digestive. Included among these are emotional stress or upset, certain endocrinopathies (e.g., panhypopituitarism), vitamin deficiency (e.g., thiamine), and certain drugs. Furthermore, depending on the nature of the responsible factors, anorexia may vary in duration from transient and short-lived to prolonged and persistent.

"**E**arly satiety *is full gratification of appetite by a small amount of food.*"

Clinical Implications

The physician who sets out to unravel the cause and significance of impaired appetite in a given patient is best advised to ascertain first that food intake is indeed impaired and truly the result of loss of "appetite." Having established to his or her satisfaction that both of these are indeed the case, the physician should then look for clues to possible causes in the physical examination of the patient. Should none be found, and should the anorexia be more than transient in duration, a directed search for a cause must be made using various diagnostic approaches. With respect to the digestive tract, the search should be all the more exacting if there are such concurrent symptoms as weight loss, nausea, vomiting, abdominal pain, diarrhea, newly developed constipation, or gastrointestinal bleeding. In such clinical settings, anorexia has an ominous ring and is a diagnostically demanding symptom. To be noted in this regard is that anorexia, with or without recognized weight loss, may exist for some time before a serious organic digestive disease, such as cancer, becomes apparent.

The disorders from which anorexia must principally be distinguished also have certain implications that merit comment. Anorexia, sitophobia, and early satiety may on occasion be present concomitantly, but each has its own implication and clinical significance.

Should the history of a patient complaining of impaired appetite disclose that the problem actually is that of sitophobia rather than anorexia, the causes of discomfort of this nature need to be sought. Prominent among the several etiologic factors demanding consideration would be an ulcerative lesion of the upper gastrointestinal tract. Another is impaired mesenteric arterial circulation, especially in an older person with evidence of cardiovascular disease, such as coronary insufficiency expressed by angina pectoris, or inadequate peripheral arterial circulation manifested by intermittent claudication.

If careful questioning establishes that the impaired eating pattern and likely associated weight loss (see Chapter 7, "Weight Loss") arose out of a feeling of being stuffed after barely beginning a meal (*early satiety*), primary suspicion should be directed at some disorder diminishing the capacity of the stomach or its ability to distend in accommodation to the intake of solid food and liquids. Linitis plastica arising from a submucosal spreading cancer of the stomach, diffuse fibrotic inflammation of the stomach wall affecting distensibility, or a large, space-occupying lesion are possible causes.

> *"Anorexia may exist for some time before an organic digestive disorder becomes clinically apparent."*

Illustrative Case

A 72-year-old man is seen because of a recent change in appetite and even more recent weight loss. The patient described his complaints in the following words:

> I have always been a good eater—never left anything on my plate and enjoyed every bit I ate. Over the past month, after I take just a few mouthfuls I feel stuffed and don't care to eat any more. And that goes for foods I used to like to eat. I don't have a scale and so I'm not sure about my weight, but in the past couple of weeks I've had to pull in my belt one notch. All this is strange to me and I'm worried."

When pressed further, the patient did not depart from his description of his complaints. His desire for food, even for his favorite—rare roast beef—was not as sharp as it had been most of his life. Nevertheless, he still looked forward to meals. The major change was the fullness he felt shortly after he began to eat. This destroyed what little desire he had left to eat and he found himself leaving a sizable portion of each meal on his plate, something he could not ever remember doing in the past.

His weight was about 8 pounds less than it was 6 months previously when he had last weighed himself. Physical examination otherwise was not remarkable. There was no skin or eyeball discoloration. No lymph nodes could be felt in the neck or elsewhere. No masses could be felt in the abdomen, and digital examination of the rectum disclosed only symmetric, smooth enlargement of the prostate.

It was the clinical impression that while the patient probably had some degree of anorexia, his principal distress was related to early satiety. A series of investigations predominantly of the upper gastrointestinal tract were therefore ordered. These were considered necessary because of the patient's age and the nature of his recently appearing symptoms.

Findings. A complete blood count was notable for a hemoglobin of 11.8 g per deciliter and a hematocrit of 32 percent. Barium-meal radiography showed the stomach to be smooth in outline and uniformly reduced in size. Introduction of air into the stomach did not result in any appreciable distention. The roentgenographic interpretation was linitis plastica of undetermined cause.

Gastroscopy was remarkable only for lack of discernible increase in luminal size when air was pumped into the stomach. Several biopsy samples were taken of the gastric mucosa, including one deep biopsy. A computed tomographic scan showed the gastric wall to be uniformly thickened.

All the gastric mucosal biopsies showed only normal-appearing gastric mucosa except the deep biopsy. Included in the latter was a small portion of submucosa containing cells with large nuclei and mitotic changes suspicious of carcinoma. The changes noted and the limited size of the sample, however, did not permit a certain diagnosis.

Management. Exploratory laparotomy was done. The stomach was found to be thickened, and several enlarged perigastric lymph nodes were detected. Frozen-section examination of a full-wall biopsy of the body of the stomach disclosed a submucosal spreading adenocarcinoma. Total gastrectomy with wide removal of lymph node-bearing perigastric tissue was performed. Histologic examination of fixed and stained preparations confirmed the frozen-section biopsy diagnosis of submucosal spreading adenocarcinoma.

To Sum Up

Anorexia is a frequently encountered, important symptom with multiple causes. Of fundamental importance is a clear understanding of the meaning of the term and its connotation. Anorexia must be distinguished in particular from sitophobia and early satiety, and an appreciation of the difference between appetite and hunger is vital in its distinction. Within the context of the digestive tract and its disorders, anorexia merits serious attention and appropriately directed studies aimed at its elucidation.

References

1. Haubrich WS. Medical meanings: A glossary of word origins. New York: Harcourt, Brace, Jovanovich, 1984.
2. Morley JE, Levine AS, Krahn DD. Neurotransmitter regulation of appetite and eating. In: Blinder BJ, Chaitin BF, Goldstein RS, eds. The eating disorders: Medical and psychological bases of diagnosis and treatment. New York: PMA Publishing, 1988:11–18.
3. Brobeck JR. Regulation of feeding and drinking. In: Handbook of physiology, sect. I, vol II. Neurophysiology. Washington: American Physiological Society, 1960:1197–1206.
4. Paintal AS. Regulation of food intake. In: Blinder BJ, Chaitin BF, Goldstein RS, eds. The eating disorders: Medical and psychological bases of diagnosis and treatment. New York: PMA Publishing, 1988:123–129.

EATING DISORDERS

Barton J. Blinder, M.D., Ph.D.

14

Eating disorders likely to be encountered in patients served by any clinician include anorexia nervosa, bulimia nervosa, pica, and rumination. These are emotional-behavioral syndromes with potentially severe physical consequences. In these disorders, erratic behavior centers on food—how it is selected or rejected and how it is consumed or voided or purged. Aberrant attitudes become habitual, and behavior becomes reactive; the ultimate result is adverse effects on the patient's nutritional and overall health status. Those close to the patient—family and friends—view the patient as being out of control with regard to eating. They may share a feeling that the patient is on the verge of serious physical deterioration, which indeed often is the case. The patient's provocative, oppositional, or secretive behavior gives rise to conflicts over issues of dependence, individuality, and personal autonomy.

Because the patient with this type of eating disorder almost invariably will deny or minimize the existence of a problem, the physician is obliged to rely heavily on the patient's family and friends for information pertaining to altered eating habits, skipped meals, and evidence of secretive eating or purging. Those close to the patient often have observed that the patient has become irritable, defensive, and withdrawn. More objective is information relating to comparative body weight. Weight fluctuations in the range of 10 percent are expected in bulimic patients, whereas in patients with anorexia nervosa weight loss often can be precipitous and in the range of 25 percent or more.

During adolescence and young adulthood, the perceived image of the body is very often a central concern, with consequent preoccupation with eating and weight control. Patients with restrictive anorexia nervosa relentlessly pursue "thinness" as a perfectionistic goal, at the same time denying the consequences of malnutrition. Bulimic patients tend to be preoccupied with bodily dissatisfaction, thus justifying their binging and purging.

> *"The patient with an eating disorder tends to deny or minimize the existence of a problem."*

The physician must become informed not only about current or recent preceding events in the patient's history, but also about the patient's developmental history. Careful inquiry must be made about eating disturbances in infancy and childhood and about any family history of eating disorders that may differ from that of the patient but may be significant nonetheless.

> *"The perceived image of the body is often a central concern."*

Anorexia Nervosa

The essence of anorexia nervosa, as stated, is an unrelenting pursuit of thinness, encountered most often in adolescent girls and young women. This is achieved by the patient principally by purposeful avoidance of eating by overt or by devious means. The patient experiences an unreasonable, yet intense, fear of weight or becoming "fat."

Sir William Gull, the English physician who provided the classic description of anorexia nervosa in the late nineteenth century, commented on the typical patient's willful refusal to eat, the denial of illness, and an insistence to be "on the move" despite physical emaciation.

The clinician can expect the patient to present innumerable rationalizations for limiting food intake. For example, the patient may point to the risk of known or unknown additives or preservatives in prepared food items, or there may be complaints of postprandial bloating and a disturbed feeling of fullness, even after consuming only a morsel of food. At the same time, the patient, when questioned diligently but tolerantly, will report unusually strenuous physical activity, such as several hours of daily exercise or calisthenics. Performance in schoolwork may appear to be maintained, but on close questioning, often the physician will find that studying is done less efficiently and that cognition, formerly acute, has become dulled.

Weight loss greater than 15 percent and failure to gain weight expected in the course of normal adolescent growth are two of the criteria for anorexia

> "*P*atients with anorexia nervosa offer innumerable rationalizations for limiting food intake."

nervosa. Other symptoms and signs that are almost invariably present include persistent amenorrhea (3 months or longer), abnormally delayed onset of menstruation, musculoskeletal pain, intolerance of cold, bradycardia, palpitation, hypotension, dry skin, brittle hair and nails, the appearance of lanugo (downy hair on the face and body), dental deterioration, and muscle wasting.

The family may report that the patient has become unusually finicky about eating or often fails to appear at mealtime. The observed quantity of food consumed is markedly reduced, especially of fats and sweets. At the same time,

> "*E*ating slowly, cutting food into small pieces, aimlessly moving food around the plate, and hiding unconsumed food are common practices."

the patient may eat inordinate amounts of vegetables and may use noncaloric condiments in excess. Family members may have observed the patient to eat exceedingly slowly, to cut food into minute pieces, and to aimlessly move bits of food around the plate. Often the patient will try to hide unconsumed food or discard food from the plate when the attention of others at the table is diverted.

In addition to the distortion of body image and aberrant eating behavior, the patient frequently exhibits obsessional rigidity, perfectionism, and aloofness. Expression of emotions often is blunted, and the ability to label or communicate feelings is limited. The physician may detect overt depression and anxiety, particularly (and perhaps unexpectedly) as nutrition improves.

Rejection of sexuality and avoidance of the demands of maturity often lead to family conflicts and tend to keep the patient socially isolated. If the anorexic is a young married woman, her spouse is likely to become puzzled and frustrated by his wife's health-endangering behavior, libidinal withdrawal, and infertility.

Illustrative Case

A 17-year-old girl, a senior in high school, was noted by her family and friends to be losing weight over a period of 4 months. She aggressively pursued aerobic exercises and walked and jogged several miles a day. At home she often avoided meals and was noted to eat slowly. She had also progressively narrowed the variety of foods she consumed to the point where she ate few foods other than those considered to be "low calorie." She was irritable, occasionally tearful, and had become more and more socially withdrawn.

When questioned, the patient denied any eating problems but did complain of feeling bulky in parts of her body (thighs, abdomen, buttocks). Examination disclosed that she had lost over 15 percent of her body weight and had a low pulse rate. Further inquiry uncovered cold intolerance, fatigue, loss of pleasurable sensations (anhedonia), and missed menses over the previous 3 months.

The patient described frequent arguments with her parents over her restriction of food intake. She stated that she had become emotionally paralyzed and indecisive in response to her "intrusive" parents. The patient's family, on the other hand, was puzzled over her denial of any problem related to food, her rigidly restrictive eating behavior, and her seeming indifference to her physical and mental deterioration. All these changes contrasted sharply with the "ideal child" and delightful teenager she had been.

Comment. This patient shows the denial of illness and gradually encroaching weight loss that are typical of anorexia nervosa. Her present severely self-destructive behavior made her a totally different person from the almost angelic child the family knew previously. The amenorrhea and pronounced body weight loss she experienced are objective anchor points in the diagnosis of this eating disorder.

Bulimia

Descriptions of bulimia, or "binge-eating," can be found in ancient writings. In the Talmud, reference is made to *boolmut,* a hyperphagic disorder occurring in emotionally troubled persons. The Greek word *boulimia,* meaning "excessive hunger," is derived from *bous* (ox) and *limos* (hunger); the Greeks commonly alluded to anything huge or monstrous as being "like an ox." In ancient Rome, binging and subsequent regurgitation were an accepted social ritual at banquets and feasts. In the nineteenth century, there were reports of "epidemics" of hysterical binging and vomiting in female boarding schools. Contrary to the popular view, bulimia is not new.

Accepted criteria for the diagnosis of bulimia nervosa include:

1. Recurring episodes of binge-eating (defined as rapid consumption of large amounts of food in discrete periods of time, usually less than 2 hours).
2. At least 3 of the following:
   a. Consumption of high-calorie, easily ingested food during a binge.
   b. Attempts to eat inconspicuously during a binge.
   c. Termination of binges by abdominal pain, sleep, or social interruption, or by self-induced vomiting.
   d. Repeated attempts to lose weight by severely restricted dieting, self-induced vomiting, or use of cathartics or diuretics.
   e. Frequent fluctuations in weight exceeding 10 pounds, because of alternating binges and fasts.

Patients with bulimia nervosa are aware that their eating patterns are abnormal and they fear not being able to stop eating. They also exhibit a depressed mood with self-deprecatory thoughts following binges.

Often the patient initially will deny all aspects of the disorder. Self-induced vomiting may eventually be admitted, but more often this is discovered or inferred by family members who find concealed vomitus stored in bags, a pervasive odor of vomitus, a telltale ring around the toilet bowl, or concealed emetics, such as ipecac.

---

*"**B**inge-eating episodes occur on the average about 10 times a week."*

Binges may occur as often as 10 times a day, although the average frequency is approximately 10 times a week.

The physician should inquire about the use (or abuse) of laxatives, diuretics, and emetics. The abuse of such agents is a sign of "counterweight" or "purgative" behavior that fosters the fantasy of "cleansing" oneself and counteracting the caloric "fattening" effect of food. The intensity of the compulsion to binge and then purge may lead to irrational hoarding of food or to a reckless kleptomania for food. On further inquiry, the patient may admit spending an entire day driving from store to store or from restaurant to restaurant, stashing bags of food (or vomitus) in her car.

Binges usually occur outside of normal mealtimes and when the patient is alone, as in the early morning, late afternoon, or middle of the night. Incredible quantities of carbohydrates, sweets, and easily prepared high-calorie foods—many in the "junk food" category—are consumed in surprisingly brief periods. If the patient can be persuaded to describe her binges, she will admit to gulping her food with no subjective sense of satiety until she feels discomforting abdominal distention. Consumption may range from 2,000 to 20,000 calories in one sitting. When a binge is not terminated by vomiting, it may be followed by protracted anorexia.

The bulimic patient may relate that her binges were triggered by acute feelings of anxiety, depression, loneliness, detachment, and isolation. Often she may recall vivid memories of childhood conflicts with rejecting or overly intrusive parents. A family history of alcoholism and physical or sexual abuse also may be described.

"Binges usually occur outside normal meal times."

Patients with bulimia nervosa appear to rebel against limitations of what others regard as rational and healthy eating. There is a peculiar sense of pseudo-satisfaction through asserting "self-control" by purging the body of both food and "negative feelings." Some patients describe experiencing the recapitulation of an earlier sense of security or mastery through their bulimic behavior. The psychologic profile of these patients frequently includes anxiety, depression, impulsive behavior (including sexual promiscuity and chemical dependency), and low self-esteem.

Among the more objective symptoms and signs are those associated with hypokalemia (induced by vomiting and laxative abuse), hypoproteinemia (despite normal body weight), parotid gland swelling (often accompanied by increased serum salivary isoamylase activity), skin erosions on the dorsal surface of the hand (from abrasion by the teeth during self-induced vomiting), corrosion of the lingual surface of the teeth (from regurgitated gastric acid), iron deficiency anemia, and oligomenorrhea or amenorrhea. Other complications that have been noted include subconjunctival hemorrhage induced by retching, peripheral neuropathy, occult spinal fractures due to osteoporosis, and gastric rupture.

Illustrative Case

A 21-year-old college junior was noted by her family to have become withdrawn and irritable. Remnants of food were found in her dormitory room, and often she absented herself from usual dinner meals. When the patient appeared at the student health clinic complaining of swollen parotid glands, laboratory examination revealed a serum potassium level of 2.7 mEq per liter as well as lowered carbon dioxide and chloride values. Confronted with these findings and the possible explanation for them, the patient tearfully admitted to being "out of control" with a chaotic eating schedule.

She also described binging almost daily on high-calorie carbohydrates (cookies, doughnuts, and bread) followed by self-induced vomiting. She was becoming desperate and feared "blowing up like a balloon" (she had in fact gained 5 pounds in the past 6 months since the behavior began). Further discussion revealed that the patient had feelings of stress because of the competitive atmosphere at school, both academically and socially. She also confided that she secretly admired her fashionably trim female peers, who seemed to succeed effortlessly in maintaining their physical appearance.

As a teenager, the patient has been of normal weight and had a "full figure." She was socially active and dated. However, she now recalled subtle remarks by friends encouraging her to "lose a little weight."

Comment. The futile, chaotic pattern of eating and the disruptive social behavior seen in bulimia are well illustrated by this patient. In those disposed to this disorder, a restrained eating pattern for the purpose of weight loss may expand into hyperphagic bouts, a mixed-up eating schedule, and a feeling of personal incompetence. Physical alterations and imbalanced laboratory values related to the nutritional impairment imposed by the bizarre eating habits of these patients are common findings.

Pica

Pica is a pathologic craving for and consequent eating of (1) substances not commonly regarded as food or, (2) of an oddly selected single food item. Examples of the first category include ice (pagophagia), clay (geophagia),

---

"Pica is most often associated with, and probably caused by, deficiency in body iron stores."

---

laundry starch (amylophagia), paper (papyrophagia), and ashes (cautopyreiophagia). Foods commonly found in the second category include pickles, olives, raw potato, and plant leaves or seeds.

Pica is most often associated with, and is probably caused by, deficiency in body iron stores. In many cases, pica disappears promptly when iron content is restored. Pica also has been associated with diets deficient in zinc and calcium. Among other proffered causes of pica are vestigial instinct, ethnic tradition, and superstition. The disorder frequently occurs during pregnancy.

In children 18 to 36 months of age, pica may be observed as an almost normal variant of behavior that is usually outgrown. Physicians serving institutions caring for the mentally retarded can expect to encounter the disorder with unusual frequency. It may also be found in coexistence with anorexia, hyperphagia, or rumination.

A complication of pica is the formation of bezoars (concretions in the alimentary canal) as a result of accumulation in the stomach of swallowed hair (trichobezoar) or undigestible plant cellulose (phytobezoar). Trichobezoars typically occur in persons with obsessional or delusional disorders. Trichotillomania is a compulsion to pull out hair, which often is then swallowed.

Other complications include dental injury, gastric or intestinal obstruction, rectal impaction (frequently found in children who eat sand or dirt), and parasitosis.

Pica is more often discovered by observant family members or friends, or incidental to the finding of iron-deficiency anemia, than by a voluntary admission from the patient. The perspicacious physician often can elicit a history of pica by inquiring gently about unusual cravings. Frequently, the patient is relieved to learn that such bizarre behavior has been recognized in others. In cases of associated iron deficiency, the patient will be further reassured when informed that the condition can be treated effectively.

☐ *Illustrative Case*

A 58-year-old married woman, in apparent good general health, had developed the strange habit, over the previous 4 months, of ingesting several trays of ice cubes daily (pagophagia). She had also noted a desire to eat small, raw potatoes (geomelophagia). Closer questioning revealed that she had noted mild fatigue while doing housework and some breathlessness when climbing stairs.

Laboratory examinations showed a hemoglobin count of 9.8 g per deciliter and a serum iron level of 30 mg per deciliter. Occult blood was present in the stool. Barium enema disclosed a carcinoma of the ascending colon.

Comment. Pica may appear spontaneously in otherwise emotionally well-adjusted patients in response to anemia and depletion of body iron stores. The latter may result from occult or protracted blood loss secondary to undiscovered neoplasm or, on occasion, bleeding from the genital tract. Laboratory studies, as was true in this patient, may reveal decreased serum iron and hemoglobin values. The iron depletion leads to decreased central nervous system dopamine neurotransmission, which may be related to the mechanisms governing food selection.

Rumination

Rumination is the regurgitation of food from the stomach back into the throat and mouth, often followed by re-chewing and re-swallowing. The term is derived from the Latin *ruminare,* meaning "to chew the cud." Merycism, a term of Greek origin, was used in early literature to denote rumination. Ruminating behavior has been observed from infancy through adulthood.

In infants, an underlying defect may be a congenital hiatus hernia; in adults there may be an abnormally obtuse angle of entry of the esophagus into the stomach or impaired lower esophageal sphincter tone (see Chapter 3, "Heartburn").

In adolescents, rumination may be a concomitant feature of other eating disorders, notably anorexia nervosa and bulimia nervosa, or it may occur as an alimentary expression of anxiety or depression.

Rumination in adults tends to be a chronically aberrant behavior. The act of bringing gastric content into the mouth appears almost involuntary, seemingly effortless, and is not preceded by nausea. The occurrence of rumination may be hidden in complaints of belching, nonspecific dyspeptic complaints, or halitosis. Adult ruminators usually try to conceal their habit and are unlikely to volunteer the symptom.

"Rumination may be hidden in complaints of belching, 'indigestion,' or halitosis."

To determine the presence of rumination, the patient must be questioned extensively and perceptively. The physician must be especially alert to complications that can be the consequence of this seemingly benign behavior. Among the more serious of these are aspiration pneumonia, electrolyte disorders, dehydration, and, in the infant, failure to thrive.

Illustrative Case

A 14-year-old girl had become depressed, withdrawn, and prone to oppositional behavior 2 months after the suicide of her college-aged brother. She complained that food frequently regurgitated into her mouth and had to be re-chewed and re-swallowed. Her grief over the loss of her brother was masked by an intense desire to be with her girlfriends; she also had an underlying sense of guilt for having concealed from her parents her brother's depression and suicidal thoughts.

Physical examination was unrevealing. Barium-meal radiography showed that, after swallowing, the gastric contents repeatedly regurgitated freely to the mouth, where they were temporarily retained, and then re-chewed and re-swallowed. All other studies were unremarkable.

Comment. Ruminatory behavior may appear in adolescents in response to bereavement. The patient described here showed a ruminatory response following her brother's death by suicide, a tragic event that for her was not only a severe loss but also filled her with guilt. Depression and detachment of the mother may lead to ruminatory behavior in an infant. Such ruminatory responses may represent a reactive pattern related to neuroendocrine deficits associated with depression and detachment.

To Sum Up

Disordered eating habits, even the most egregious, have a venerable history going back to ancient times; only recently, however, have they gained popular and, indeed, proper medical recognition. Patients suffering from these disorders are notoriously reticent to discuss their symptoms and often go to great lengths to conceal their aberrant behavior. Only by being aware of the problems involved and perspicacious in the phrasing of questions can the physician gain the full picture, thus permitting the prospect of effective treatment.

Suggested Reading

Blinder BJ. Developmental antecedents of the eating disorders: A reconsideration. Psych Clin North Am 1980; 3:579–592.

Blinder BJ. Rumination: A benign disorder? Int J Eating Dis 1986; 5:385–386.

Blinder BJ, Bain N, Simpson R. Evidence for an opioid neurotransmission mechanism in adult rumination. Am J Psych 1986; 143:255.

Blinder BJ, Cadenhead K. Bulimia: A historical overview. Adolescent Psych 1986; 13:231–240.

Blinder BJ, Chaitin BF, Goldstein R. The eating disorders: Medical and psychological bases of diagnosis and treatment. New York: PMA Publishing, 1988.

Blinder BJ, Hagman J. Serum salivary isoamylase in anorexia nervosa, bulimia or bulimia nervosa. Hillside J Clin Psych 1986; 8:152–163.

Wu JC, Hagman JO, Buchsbaum MS, et al. Greater left cerebral hemispheric metabolism in bulimia assessed by positron emission tomography. Am J Psych 1990; 147:309–312.

DISTURBED ORAL AND NASAL SENSATIONS

William S. Haubrich, M.D.

15

Because the mouth and nose are intimately associated with alimentary function, both physiologically and pathologically as well as in the minds of many patients, symptoms referable to diminished or distorted oral or nasal sensations often are commingled with various digestive complaints. Occasionally an oral or nasal symptom may be the presenting problem. Among these common complaints are impaired or distorted taste and smell, sore mouth and tongue, and bad breath (halitosis). These symptoms may sometimes seem trivial to the physician but often they are distressing to the patient. Always, they deserve thoughtful attention.

In most cases, the cause of altered taste or smell sensations can be closely approximated, if not established, by information provided by the patient. Often, a perceptive history can lead to an effective remedy.

Altered Taste and Smell

Although the sense of taste and smell are anatomically distinct, they are often symptomatically confused. What many people call "taste" is really "flavor," and flavor is a combination of both taste and smell. Even when taste is separated from smell, the implied sense is not alone the four basic perceptions of salty, sour, sweet, and bitter; it also includes the oral tactile feeling of texture and temperature. Most patients who complain "I've lost my taste" will be found to have a diminished or absent olfactory sense. In some conditions, both smell and taste can be impaired. Isolated loss of taste sensation alone is relatively

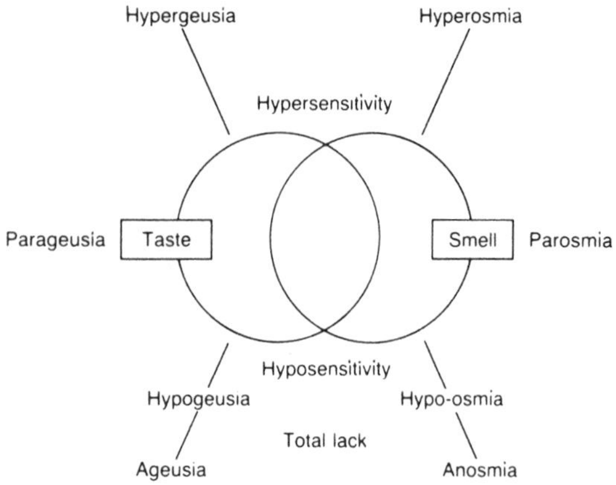

Hypergeusia   Hyperosmia

Hypersensitivity

Parageusia   Taste   Smell   Parosmia

FIGURE 15-1. Aberrations in taste and
smell. (Reprinted with permission from
Haubrich WS. Other symptoms encountered
in gastroenterologic practice. In: Berk JE,
Haubrich WS, Kalser MH, Roth JLA,
Schaffner F, eds. Bockus Gastroenterology.
4th ed. Philadelphia: WB Saunders,
1985:193.

Hyposensitivity
Hypogeusia   Hypo-osmia
Total lack
Ageusia   Anosmia

infrequent. In elderly persons, the acuity of both taste and smell tends to diminish as part of the natural aging process.

The various designations of aberrations in taste and smell are illustrated in Figure 15–1. The usual impairment is that of diminished sensation; total abolition of either taste or smell is less frequent. Relatively few patients complain of disturbingly heightened sensitivity (although some husbands have been known to lament their wives' alleged hyperbolic reactions to barely perceptible odors). Especially strange are the distorted or bizarre perceptions of taste and smell (*parageusia* and *parosmia*) in which the patient is fully aware of a given stimulus but describes the sensation in terms far from normal. Also in this category are *phantogeusia* and *phantosmia,* perceptions of taste or odor for which there is no appropriate stimulus.

How to Inquire About Altered Taste and Smell

The answers to a few simple and obvious questions will help to tell whether taste or smell, or a combination of both, is at fault. Questions should be directed to perceptions of familiar substances. A response to "How does coffee taste to you?" may indicate that the patient is well aware the coffee he or she sips is liquid and warm, and sweet if taken with sugar, but the statement "It doesn't have any flavor" suggests that the problem is olfactory. A response such as "I know it has the flavor of coffee, but the sugar doesn't make it sweet" suggests a defect in taste. Another question might be "Can you tell the difference between vanilla and chocolate ice cream?" The response "Both are sweet and smooth, but otherwise they taste the same" indicates olfactory impairment. Inability to perceive salty and sweet tastes suggests a lingual lesion, such as lichen planus, or a facial nerve (cranial nerve VII) lesion. Diminished sour and bitter tastes suggest a palatal problem, as in edentulous patients obliged to wear an upper dental plate.

Further inquiry can reveal whether impairment is partial or complete. Sharply contrasting foods or odors may be distinguished easily, but the capacity to distinguish subtle differences between similar substances may be lost.

The physician may ask the patient: Is impairment of taste or smell total or partial? Is perception too weak or too strong? Is perception of taste or smell of some things retained while that of others is lost? Do certain things taste or smell differently than before? Is impairment unilateral or bilateral, that is, can odors be perceived when inhaling through one nostril but not the other, and do substances seem to taste the same on either side of the mouth?

"Questions should be directed to perception of familiar substances."

Onset and Duration of Impairment.   The onset and duration of impairment may give a clue to the cause. A sudden loss of taste or smell suggests a precipitous provocation. The most frequent cause, as everyone knows, is the "common cold." With simple colds, the problem may be merely an effusion of mucus that insulates the nasal membranes; when the mucus clears, sensation is regained. However, there are viral infections of the nasal passages that can actually injure the olfactory receptors and their afferent pathways. In such cases, impairment can last for weeks or months after apparent recovery from the inciting infection. The onset of uremia may be marked by diminished sensitivity of taste and smell. Another cause of abrupt impairment is head injury, especially that associated with "concussion" or followed by amnesia for the event. If both taste and smell are lost, was it simultaneously? Or did the loss of one sense precede the loss of the other? The answers may help determine the location and extent of the lesion.

Has the Loss Been Unremitting or Variable?   Occasionally, the acuity of a sense will vary. If this is so, is there a diurnal pattern (suggesting hormonal influence) or a relation to ambience (suggesting environmental conditions, possibly pollutants)? Constant exposure to pungent odors can result in an adaptive hyposmia, although after removal of the stimulus the sense is rapidly regained. In some cases, curiously, even in the absence of the stimulus the perception of a particular odor lingers or recurs. In premenopausal women, olfaction is said to be keener about the time of ovulation and less sensitive during menses. Is there seasonal variation (suggesting a role of allergy or exposure to air-conditioning or to winter heating and low humidity)? Over time, has the loss become greater, stayed the same, or lessened?

Preceding Medical Events. An account of preceding medical events can be revealing. In addition to noting previous allergic diathesis, inquiry should be directed to more immediate infections, particularly of the upper respiratory tract. Mention has been made that loss of taste and smell can persist long after nasopharyngeal infection has seemed to clear. Other systemic infections may be implicated. Viral hepatitis, even that occurring in the absence of icterus, is known to confer a marked and unaccustomed aversion to a taste for tobacco and alcohol, as well as for common foods; the aversion usually disappears when infection subsides.

Impairment or distortion of taste may be an early symptom complex of otherwise occult malignancy, particularly cancers in the lung, ovary, and breast. A long-held belief is that distaste for meat is a sign of gastric carcinoma.

Previous surgical procedures, especially those requiring inhalant anesthesia, should be noted. Of particular concern are procedures directed to the head and neck. Why were they undertaken? Precisely what was done? Inquiry should be made about preceding dental disorders or manipulations, including the application of dental prostheses.

Medications. A detailed account of all medications recently or currently taken may give a clue to the cause of the problem. Numerous drugs have been implicated in alteration of taste and smell. Some ingested or injected drugs or their metabolites (e.g., tetracycline, ethambutol, biguanide, penicillamine, and allopurinol) are actually excreted in saliva resulting in the peculiar sensation often described as "a metallic taste." Some drugs tend to distort normal taste (e.g., sulfasalazine, metronidazole, tegretol, and nifedipine). Other drugs impair taste by suppressing the flow of saliva, thus inducing a dry mouth (e.g., anticholinergic agents, certain antihistamines, and most tricyclic antidepressants).

> **"A** detailed account of all medications recently or currently taken may give a clue to the cause of impaired taste."

Review of Systems. An orderly review of systems can be revealing. Aside from impaired taste or smell, has there been nasal congestion or discharge? Has breathing been impeded? Is the patient aware of unaccustomed mouth-breathing? Does the flow of saliva seem diminished? Complaints of impaired or disagreeable taste are frequent in patients exhibiting a sicca syndrome, such as encountered in various collagen-vascular diseases.

Neurologic disorders that may be implicated include temporal lobe epilepsy, Korsakoff's psychosis, parkinsonism, and Alzheimer's disease. The cranial neoplasm most frequently associated with impaired olfaction is meningioma.

Altered Diet Patterns.   Particular attention should be directed to dietary patterns and symptoms of alimentary dysfunction. Loss of taste or smell can be both a cause and an effect of nutritional deficiency. An egregious dietary idiosyncrasy or restriction may have led to deficiency in vitamins or trace metals, notably zinc and copper. Impaired nutritional assimilation, especially that due to pancreatic exocrine insufficiency, has been associated with loss of taste and smell.

Inherited Defects.   The possibility of an inherited defect can be explored by inquiring about the family history. Certain genetically transmitted syndromes have been described in which impairment in taste and smell is associated with other defects, such as alopecia, deafness, and hypogonadism. Nasal polyposis, in some cases, can be a familial trait.

Personal Habits.   Finally, the patient's personal habits will have to be taken into account. It is common knowledge that smoking tobacco dulls and distorts the senses of both taste and smell. The use of snuff or chewing tobacco has an even more damaging effect. Potentially most injurious is the sniffing of cocaine, formerly an exotic recreation but now, regrettably, a commonplace habit. More subtle and less often appreciated is the suppression of taste sensitivity by chronic alcohol imbibition. Doubtless this contributes to the nutritional neglect so commonly seen in alcoholics.

Dysgeusia.   Distinct from the problem of reduced capacity for appreciating the sensation of taste is the complaint of disagreeable taste (*dysgeusia*). This is usually described by the patient as simply "a bad taste in the mouth." Some patients, on further questioning, can distinguish their disagreeable taste sensation as "sour," "bitter," "cloyingly sweet," "always salty," or "metallic." Many will say only that their taste is "foul." The key question then becomes "Is the bad or foul taste always there or does it come and go?" In the latter case, attention should be directed to discovering a specific precipitating cause, which might be the use of a particular medication. A foul taste temporarily relieved by a mouthwash is likely to be caused by stagnant saliva or the exudate of periodontal disease.

More often the patient will complain that the bad taste is "always there." This is curious because normally perceived taste is adaptable—that is, the sensation wanes even when the stimulating substance remains. Unremitting bad or bitter taste is a strong indication of an underlying neurotic disorder, usually a depressed state. It is not mere coincidence that in our everyday language the word "taste" is used in both an objective and a figurative sense. One might be said to have "poor taste," meaning impaired oral sensation, commonly, however, "poor taste" is a pejorative assertion of faulty judgment or attitude. For many patients complaining of unremitting bad or bitter taste this may be an expression of "organ language," whereby the sufferer is really saying "Something is wrong, something is not as it should be."

Examining the Patient

What can be expected to be seen in the mouth of the typical patient complaining of a bad taste? One searches, of course, for evidence of poor dental hygiene, periodontal disease, fouled dentures, or a heavily coated tongue, but such obvious explanations are not often encountered. Rather, the oral cavity usually will appear relatively normal. (The sometimes startling appearance of a "geographic tongue" usually is not associated with impaired taste.) More often than not, a complaint of bad taste by a patient who has a fairly clean mouth is a symptom of depression. A few simple questions should furnish supporting evidence with the patient's admission of jaded appetite, unprovoked fatigue, ennui, inability to concentrate, and delayed insomnia. Although hardly a therapeutic test, a prescription of antidepressive medication (other than tricyclic compounds) often alleviates the sensation of bad taste. It is rarely helpful to refer a patient with a clean mouth to a dentist in the hope of eradicating some occult cause of the complaint.

In cases of disturbed olfactory sensation, the obvious place to look is the nose; however, in the absence of nasal obstruction, heavy exudate, grossly abnormal nasal membranes or polyposis, not much will be apparent. Subtler changes may be evident to an experienced rhinologist.

A comprehensive physical examination occasionally will reveal findings suggestive of conditions mentioned previously in "Review of Systems." Absence of physical abnormalities will be reassuring to both the patient and the physician, making a complete examination worthwhile.

> "'**B**ad taste,' more often than not, is a symptom of depression."

Objective testing of taste and smell can be undertaken, but unless such tests are conducted by an expert, the results are difficult to interpret and often may be misleading. It is helpful to know that there are specialized clinics for the investigation and treatment of taste and smell disorders in many medical centers.*

*Among these are specially equipped and staffed centers at the University of Connecticut, State University of New York at Syracuse, University of Pennsylvania in Philadelphia, University of Cincinnati, and University of Colorado in Denver.

Illustrative Case

A 62-year-old housewife was referred by an oral surgeon with the request that the alimentary tract be thoroughly searched for a cause of the patient's long-standing complaint of "a foul taste in the mouth." The dentist had found no lesion in the patient's oral cavity but nevertheless had prescribed a broad assortment of mouthwashes, supplemented by large doses of most known vitamins and minerals, all to no avail. The woman allowed that the sense of disagreeable taste would come and go, but she was at a loss to explain how or why. She denied feeling depressed, yet when questioned specifically, she forthrightly admitted that she was occasionally troubled by loss of appetite, an utter lack of energy despite no exertion, and withdrawal from activities she usually found engrossing. Seldom did she have difficulty in falling asleep, but often she awakened during the night for no apparent reason, only to "toss and turn" until she drowsed off again.

Her oral surgeon had repeatedly scrutinized her teeth, gums, oral mucosa, and tongue, yet no abnormality had been detected. Complete physical examination confirmed an overall healthy state. Urinalysis, hemogram, and a panel of blood chemistry tests (SMA-24) yielded no deviation from normal.

Rather than embark on a series of probably futile, invasive examinations of the alimentary canal, it was decided, after the circumstances were explained to the patient, to prescribe a nontricyclic antidepressant medication. Within a week the patient reported improvement, and after 3 weeks the bad taste had disappeared, along with most of the other symptoms of depression. At follow-up a year later the patient stated that she had learned to surmount her "blues" and had remained well.

Comment.   This case of "bad taste" was more easily explained and reme-died than many. All that was required was knowing that a disagreeable taste sensation can be a manifestation of depression, asking a few pointed questions to substantiate altered mood, and assuring the patient that her mouth was clean and her health well-maintained. She was fortunate in being among those responding rapidly to antidepressant medication.

To Sum Up

Disturbances in the senses of taste and smell are common; they are some-times presented as sole complaints but often are associated with symptoms of other diseases. In many cases, an accurate diagnosis can be postulated and an explanation arrived at by a carefully taken history and the appropriate physical examination. Patients with more difficult problems can benefit by referral to a center specializing in diagnosis and treatment of these often vexing disorders.

Sore or Burning Mouth or Tongue

Often symptomatically allied with a disturbed sense of taste is a sense of soreness or burning in the mouth or tongue. (See Table 15–1 for a summary of causes of a sore mouth or tongue.) As a rule and paradoxically, it will be found that serious lesions of the mouth or tongue are seldom painful, and painful conditions, aside from the discomfort, are seldom serious. No visible lesion is likely to be evident in the mouth of the patient complaining of a burning tongue, whereas the examiner who seeks to find an early oral cancer is usually given no clue by the patient but must rely on his or her own keen senses of vision and touch.

"Serious lesions are seldom painful, whereas painful conditions are seldom serious."

Pain in the teeth or gums, particularly when aggravated by cold liquids, almost certainly indicates dental or periodontal disease. Acute gingivitis in a previously healthy young person arouses a suspicion of acute leukemia, particularly of the myelogenous or monocytic type. Chronic or recurring gingivitis, with sore, inflamed, and swollen gums, usually is nonspecific and reflects deterioration due to neglected dental hygiene. Gingivitis resulting from vitamin deficiency, as in scurvy, is extremely rare, at least in developed countries.

Pain not in the mouth but referred to the region of the zygomatic arch, and aggravated by chewing, points to temporomandibular joint disorder. Undue fatigue while chewing indicates a defect in the muscles of mastication.

TABLE 15–1. A Checklist of Some Causes of Sore Mouth and Tongue

- Anxiety, depression, cancerophobia
- Menopausal syndrome
- Dental or denture trauma
- Tabagism, alcoholism
- Dry mouth
- Nutritional deficiency
- Aphthous stomatitis, including that of sprue
- Oral mucosal infection
- Diabetes mellitus
- Vasculitis

Glossopharyngeal neuralgia is a rare variation of tic douloureux and can involve elements of cranial nerves V, IX, and X. Paroxysms of lancinating pain occur in the tongue and throat, often extending to the ear and neck, and sometimes attended by marked slowing of the heartbeat and occasionally by syncope. No superficial lesion is visible. A clue to the diagnosis is the finding of focal trigger points by gently probing the oropharyngeal mucosa.

Scrutiny of the mouth and its contents may disclose oral lesions of which the patient is symptomatically unaware. Most common among incidentally discovered "white lesions" are those appearing in linear array opposite the level of molar occlusion. These are the result of acute or chronic dental trauma. Similar signs of inadvertent biting may be seen along the lateral margins of the tongue. When seen on the tip or along the sides of the tongue, such an appearance suggests that a swollen tongue has gotten in the way of biting, as can occur in certain forms of infiltrating disease.

Also commonly seen are Fordyce's spots, appearing as tiny, yellow, seedlike implants of engorged sebaceous glands in the buccal mucosa. Lichen planus and leukoplakia appear as pearly gray or white patches on the tongue or oral mucosa. All of these lesions are usually asymptomatic and benign, except for leukoplakia, which can be a precursor of squamous cell carcinoma.

The most common acute, focal ulceration that is painful—other than that produced by inadvertently biting the tongue or cheek—is aphthous stomatitis. Almost everyone has had experience with this pesky lesion at one time or another, yet its cause, in most cases, remains obscure. Typically the patient relates an outbreak of aphthous lesions to contracting a "cold" or suffering an "upset stomach." The sequence is predictable. The patient first feels a focal burning sensation for a day or so; then a small, superficial, painful ulcer erupts; this lasts for several days and then spontaneously disappears, usually within a week. Interestingly, the tip of the patient's tongue is keenly sensitive in detecting pre-eruptive aphthous lesions. If the lesions are not readily apparent to the examiner, the patient can be asked to point to them with his tongue, and there they will be found.

More ominous lesions, also painful, that in their early stages resemble aphthous stomatitis, are those of Behçet's syndrome and Wegener's granulomatosis. Fortunately these conditions, which represent forms of vasculitis, probably of errant immune origin, are rare. In addition to ulcerated lesions elsewhere in the skin, the visceral mucosa can be involved, resulting in abdominal pain, diarrhea, and gastrointestinal bleeding. In some cases there are symptoms and signs of widespread systemic disease, including uveitis and arthritis.

The vesicles of herpes labialis are limited to areas of mucocutaneous junction at the lips and nares. The eruption of herpes zoster, affecting the trigeminal nerve (cranial nerve V) can appear in the buccal mucosa; it is always unilateral.

Although not acutely sore, an unduly dry mouth (*xerostomia*) can be exceedingly annoying. Most often the condition is consequent to habitual mouth-breathing or the effect of drugs that suppress the flow of saliva. Such drugs include not only the familiar anticholinergics but also adrenergics, certain ganglionic blocking agents, and the tricyclic antidepressant medications. More serious is the dry mouth that is a prominent feature of the sicca complex, as in Sjögren's syndrome and various collagen-vascular diseases.

An opposite condition is *sialorrhea,* or excessive salivation, which can be a reaction to oral irritation, such as that from mucosal inflammation or ill-fitting dentures. Sialorrhea also accompanies subliminal or overt nausea. Profuse sialorrhea can lead to drooling, a symptom acceptable in infants but disdainful in adults. Drooling signifies the inability to clear saliva, from the mouth as, for example, in facial or glossopharyngeal palsy. Drooling is not only embarrassing but also can lead to painfully inflamed fissuring at the corners of the mouth (*cheilosis*). Indeed, in clinical practice, cheilosis almost always is due to drooling; rarely is it a sign of vitamin deficiency.

Glossitis (inflammation of the tongue) should be distinguished from *glossodynia* (painful tongue), although the two conditions can be concurrent. A visibly inflamed tongue usually is sore or even painful; a sore or burning tongue most often is not inflamed and appears normal.

> *"Cheilosis almost always is due to drooling; rarely is it a sign of vitamin deficiency."*

A sore and visibly reddened, smooth, or swollen tongue may be an indicator of nutritional deficiency, such as occurs in failure to take or absorb nourishment. The particular deficiency may be of iron, B-vitamins, or folate. In patients with iron deficiency, the tongue typically is smooth, pale, and lacking in muscle tone. In patients with primary pernicious anemia, the tongue may appear fiery red at the tip and lateral margins; pain tends to wax and wane. In some patients with advanced diabetes mellitus, the tongue can be beefy, red, and sore. Painless swelling of the tongue is a feature of certain forms of amyloidosis. In most cases, the symptoms of the underlying condition predominate and the tongue swelling is of minor concern to the patient.

"Geographic tongue" is striking in appearance, but usually not painful or acutely inflamed. The changing, circumscribed margins of white or yellow patches on a background of pink or red suggest a map of sea-girted islands.

Glossodynia, especially when described by the patient as "burning" (*glossopyrosis*) and in the absence of visible change in the tongue, most often is a symptom of emotional disturbance, notably depression. It is interesting that this is a complaint proffered almost exclusively by women. The typical patient is a postmenopausal woman who says that her tongue "burns" constantly, day and night. In such cases, the significance of the symptom is readily brought to light by inquiring of other common features of a depressed state. When glossodynia remits in the morning but becomes troublesome later in the day the physician should look for signs of abrasive trauma. The patient's teeth or dentures should be examined for unduly sharp edges or rough spots.

Illustrative Case

A 56-year-old postmenopausal woman was seen in the clinic because of unexplained weight loss (from her usual 140 pounds to 115 pounds within 2 years) and what she described as diarrhea. A lesser complaint was of a smooth, slightly sore tongue. She admitted that her sense of taste had become somewhat impaired; however, what she found puzzling in her loss of weight was the fact that her appetite was undiminished. She said she had been eating as much or more food than usual, a claim substantiated by her husband and daughter, who accompanied her. The looseness and frequency of her stools was variable; she denied any relationship of the stooling pattern to diet, which she said was unchanged from that she had enjoyed all of her life. When specifically questioned, she admitted being embarrassed by the extremely foul odor of her stools.

Physical examination was unrevealing except for the expected signs of weight loss and the smooth, atrophic surface of the tongue. No oral mucosal lesion or exudate was visible. Proctosigmoidoscopy showed that the mucosa was intact; however, the lumen of the sigmoid colon was filled with pasty, pale grayish-brown feces that required repeated swabbing to uncover the mucosa. The feces-soaked swabs were notably fetid.

Urinalysis was clear. The hemogram disclosed a slight, hypochromic anemia. The blood chemistry panel (SMA-24) was in the normal range, except for borderline low values for serum proteins, calcium, and cholesterol.

Upper gastrointestinal endoscopy was scheduled, not because a focal lesion was suspected but rather to permit close inspection and biopsy of the duodenum. As expected, the duodenal mucosa was intact but its surface lacked a normal, velvety, villous appearance. Three biopsy specimens were obtained. When sectioned, each showed total villous atrophy, deformity of surface epithelial cells, and excessive infiltration by lymphocytes of the lamina propria.

Comment.   This proved to be a fairly straightforward case of adult celiac disease. The "diarrhea" was readily evident as steatorrhea, both by the history and by proctosigmoidoscopy. Soreness of the tongue was a minor feature but was entirely compatible with a diagnosis of nutritional impairment.

One might have considered tests determining the serum carotene level and D-xylose excretion, a 72-hour stool collection to measure fecal fat content, and imaging the entire alimentary tract by contrast radiography. But, all of these procedures were made unnecessary by the use of endoscopic biopsy to verify the presumptive diagnosis.

A low-gluten diet was prescribed. At first the patient thought this somewhat ridiculous, insofar as she had never thought herself intolerant of gluten-containing foods. Nevertheless, she agreed to abide by the diet probably more to humor her physician than out of any faith in its benefit. To her surprise, the patient reported a prompt and favorable response. A "normal" bowel habit was resumed, she regained weight, and her usual vigor returned. She mentioned, incidentally, that she was no longer bothered by a sore tongue. After her recovery was assured, the patient confided that, before her condition was properly diagnosed, she had harbored a fear of cancer.

To Sum Up

While uncommonly an indication of a life-threatening disorder, a sore mouth or tongue can be disturbing, even to the point of unbearable distress, to the patient.

When a sore or burning tongue is the patient's sole complaint, a visible lesion is unlikely to be evident, and the symptom more often than not will be found to be an expression of a depressed state. When a sore mouth or tongue is described as part of a constellation of other symptoms or signs, a thorough review of the history and a comprehensive physical examination, supplemented by a few well-chosen laboratory or imaging procedures, usually will lead to a correct diagnosis of the underlying cause.

Bad Breath (Halitosis)

According to the clerisy of Madison Avenue, *halitosis* is a universal symptom suffered by all living creatures, requiring immediate application of whatever remedy is being touted at the moment. Like most exhortations of the advertising fraternity, the claim is somewhat exaggerated. Still, a disagreeable and offensive odor pervading the breath, however perceived, is a common complaint. Although rarely a herald of life-threatening disease, halitosis can be an almost unbearable onus to the patient.

The first concern of the clinician is to determine whether the reported bad breath is objectively or subjectively perceived—that is, whether the fetid odor is real or imagined. Have persons other than the patient remarked about the problem, or is the patient the only one aware of the odor? This is not the simple distinction it may seem. In either case, the perception is so vivid to the patient that he or she is certain that everyone must be acutely aware of the odor. If the patient is accompanied by a family member or friend, corroboration or lack thereof may be readily at hand, and the query must be put to the third party. Should the family member or friend dispute the patient's claim, it is well not to press the point (certainly not in the initial interview). If there is no available witness, one cannot, unfortunately, take the patient's word for what others may or may not have sensed. The patient with imagined halitosis will almost invariably contend "Oh, everybody knows about it."

It should be kept in mind that smell is a rapidly adaptive sense—that is, a given odor, even when pungent and persistent, is not perceived for long. The patient whose breath is truly fetid, having adapted to the odor, will often deny being aware of a stench. For the patient suffering from imagined halitosis, there is no adaptation, and the supposed awareness of the stench is constant and unremitting.

"Is 'bad breath' real or only imagined?"

There is, of course, the essential test: take a whiff of the patient's exhaled breath. This is the best and often the only method for verifying the quality of expired air (Fig. 15–2). Even this direct test is subject to error. Obviously, the clinician's own olfactory acuity must be intact and functioning. Furthermore, allowance has to be made for the fact that anyone's breath odor, foul or sweet, is not constant. Finally, the patient may have taken pains to disguise the odor. In such instances, it is not unusual to detect a distinct medicine-like breath, as if the patient has just gargled with an antiseptic solution or sucked on a deodorant lozenge. Neither is it unusual to find the patient's tongue stained green, orange,

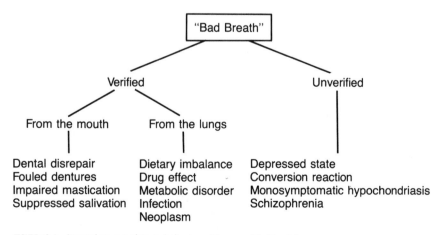

FIGURE 15–2. Suggested sequence of inquiry leading to possible causes of "bad breath."

or black from the coloring agent used in many forms of purported oral deodorants. Evidence that the patient uses breath deodorants does not distinguish between real and imagined halitosis; it does mean that the patient takes his or her complaint seriously.

Imagined Halitosis

Of the two general categories of complaint, the *idée fixe* that foul breath is exuded when, in fact, the breath is untainted, is by far less frequently encountered. Yet it is more serious and more vexing to both the patient and the physician, and, in most cases, more difficult to alleviate. The problem can be observed in four settings: (1) as an expression of a depressed state, (2) as a manifestation of conversion reaction, (3) as a monosymptomatic hypochondriasis, and (4) as a feature of schizophrenia. Which of these conditions pertains can, in large measure, be distinguished by cautious yet thorough probing of the patient's history.

Depression probably is the most common setting for imagined "bad breath," and the complaint often is accompanied by that of "bad taste in the mouth" or "sore tongue." Other well-known features of depression, such as loss of appetite, diminished capacity for concentration, ennui, decline in libido, and delayed insomnia, usually can be brought to light by means of a few gently phrased questions.

"The best test for halitosis is to smell the patient's exhaled breath."

Unverified halitosis as a conversion disorder usually is of abrupt onset and is identifiable with a precipitating circumstance; it may be of short duration, although subject to recurrence. The patient may give the impression of being indifferent to his or her plight.

Monosymptomatic hypochondriasis is the strangest and most elusive setting. The diagnosis is elusive because the delusion is projected alone; the patient's sensorium and stream of thought are otherwise intact and appropriate. Monosymptomatic hypochondriasis can take three forms: (1) a delusion that certain body parts, especially the face, despite obviously contrary evidence, are misshapen; (2) a repugnant delusion of infection, particularly by wormy parasites; and (3) an obsession with supposed emission of foul and offensive body odors, usually halitosis. In most cases, the condition is longstanding. Often the patient has been concerned with the problem long before admitting a complaint.

Unfortunately, the patient's conviction is almost unshakable. A typical remark is "No one has told me I have bad breath, but I know I do, and I know other people are offended by it." Repeated reassurance, even by persons that the patient otherwise trusts, is of little or no avail. This unfortunate patient, once the condition is identified, also will be helped best by referral to a knowledgeable and sympathetic psychotherapist.

Schizophrenia, the gravest setting, may be evident when the patient claims that the cause of the alleged malodor is being manipulated in a bizarre way from outside the patient's own body. This constitutes a paranoid olfactory hallucination. When schizophrenia is suspected, prompt referral to a psychiatrist is advised.

Verifiable Halitosis

Much more often the fetid breath is real enough and readily detected. Here the essential distinction is whether the foul odor originates in the oral cavity (*fetor ex ore*) or is in the air exhaled from the lungs. Sometimes the difference can be made evident by asking the patient to hold the nose closed and expell air from the mouth, and then compare this with the odor of air exhaled through the open nose. Another means is to sample the odor of saliva or other detritus swabbed from the mouth.

> "*An essential distinction in true halitosis is whether the foul odor originates in the oral cavity or is in air exhaled from the lungs.*"

Breath can become fetid from a variety of causes. Almost everyone knows that one's breath is hardly its sweetest when one first awakens from a night's sleep. This is normal and is usually relieved promptly by brushing the teeth and rinsing the mouth. Early morning halitosis is more troublesome for the person who habitually breathes through his or her open mouth during sleep.

The slightly acidic pH and free flow of normal saliva tend to suppress the accumulation of odor-producing bacteria in the mouth. Whatever tends to allow incubation of stagnant saliva often gives rise to the stench.

Conditions contributing to a malodorous mouth include periodontal disease or debris, soiled dental prosthetic devices, mucosal ulceration and necrosis, gingivitis, heavily coated tongue, and sparse or ropy saliva. Contributing factors may be deprivation of normal mastication (as in conditions requiring severely restricted diets), impaired motility of the tongue, deformity of the mouth (possibly iatrogenic), and palsied swallowing. The effect of medications with anticholinergic properties should also be considered.

Fetid breath arising from lower in the respiratory tract can be the result of any condition favoring an overgrowth of bacteria, especially gram-negative and anaerobic types, that liberate volatile, sulfur-containing substances by their action on proteinaceous matter. These conditions include necrotic ulcerations or neoplasms, bronchiectasis, and lung abscess. In most cases, these are predominantly symptomatic in themselves, and fetid breath is only a lesser complaint.

It is well known that the volatile essence of certain ingested substances or their metabolites, being excreted by the lungs, can impart disagreeable odors to exhaled breath. Obvious examples are garlic, onions, congeners of alcoholic beverages, and tobacco tars. Less often recognized are the odors imparted by endogenous breakdown of body fats and proteins. It has been postulated that a diet exceedingly high in fat or protein content can result in a disagreeable breath odor.

In addition to anticholinergic agents that affect saliva, other drugs can directly impart odors to the breath. The most striking example is paraldehyde, now seldom used because of this offending property. The consumer of egregious doses of vitamins, particularly those of the B group, is liable to exude a peculiar musty odor, in part coming from the breath.

Clinicians have long been familiar with sometimes distinctive breath odors of patients with uremia (described as a "mousy" odor), diabetic ketoacidosis (a sour "fruity" odor), and advanced liver disease (*fetor hepaticus*). There was a time when physicians boasted of their diagnostic acumen in distinguishing these odors; doubtless they exist, but their identifiable specificity is moot.

It might be worthwhile asking what circumstances, if any, the patient has found to alter breath odor. It may be that the patient's own olfactory perception becomes more acute, an example being the heightened sensitivity to odor experienced by some women during menses. Finally, the patient can be queried on what measures he or she has taken to allay offensive breath, and to what extent they have succeeded or failed. Almost all patients complaining of bad breath will have tried copious mouthwashes. Those with *fetor ex ore* probably will claim temporary relief; those troubled by odors emanating from the lungs will seldom report benefit; and those with imagined halitosis will adamantly deny any measure of relief.

Illustrative Case

A 28-year-old unmarried woman scheduled an appointment in the clinic because of a single complaint: "bad breath." She had taken this complaint to almost a dozen doctors in as many years, all to no avail. A dentist had referred her to the gastroenterology clinic with the suggestion, "Maybe there is something the matter with your stomach." The patient had come alone. When asked if others had made remarks about her breath, she replied, "No, no one has said anything, but I know they're bothered by it." The following dialogue then took place.

Physician: How are others bothered by your breath?
Patient: I don't know—I just know they are bothered.
Physician: Has anyone in your family said you have bad breath?
Patient: They keep telling me they can't smell it. But they're wrong. I know it's terrible. [She was on the verge of tears.]

The patient had no other complaints referable to the head, nose, or throat, or to the respiratory or alimentary tract. Her complete systems review and her past medical history were unrevealing.

At the time she was seen in the clinic she was temporarily unemployed. Since graduating from business school, she had held a number of responsible clerical jobs, but none of them for very long. She wanted to make clear she had never been fired from a job; she had always departed of her own volition. The reason was always the same: she became unbearably self-conscious about her presumably offensive breath.

Physical examination was unrevealing of any defect. Note was made that the patient's basically attractive facial features were unadorned with makeup. She wore her hair severely drawn back and knotted in a little, prim bun. She never smiled. Her voice was a monotone. Her teeth were well formed and scrupulously clean. Her tongue was tinted green; she held an oral deodorant tablet in her mouth while she was being examined. At no time, either at her initial visit or when she returned to learn the results of her tests, was any disagreeable odor detected in her exhaled breath.

Urinalysis, hemogram, and blood chemistry panel (SMA-24) were uniformly in normal ranges. A chest radiograph, recently taken elsewhere, showed clear lung fields and a normal cardiac silhouette.

The patient was persuaded, with some difficulty, that further investigation of her alimentary tract was unnecessary. When her condition was explained to her, she was offered an appointment with a psychotherapist. She protested that previous attempts at psychological evaluation had led nowhere. "They told me there was nothing wrong with me." Nevertheless, she agreed to ponder the recommendation. She never made the appointment, however, and has not returned to the clinic. Likely she continues to complain of "bad breath." One can only hope that another practitioner will be more successful in persuading her of the true nature of her problem.

Comment. This is an almost classic example of a monosymptomatic hypochondriasis. All criteria for the diagnosis were met in the initial interview and examination. Also classic, unfortunately, was the patient's rejection of the diagnosis and the recommended management. The only benefit she derived from her visit to the clinic was that she was spared, on at least that occasion, the discomfort, expense, and risk of an unnecessary series of invasive procedures.

To Sum Up

"Bad breath," whether actually fetid or only imagined to be, is seldom an alarming complaint but often can become an almost unbearable symptom to the patient. It is important to verify the offensive breath. When this has been done, the next step is to distinguish whether the origin is from the mouth or nose, the lower respiratory tract, or a systemic disorder. Most such causes can be palliated, if not cured. More vexing to both the patient and the physician is the problem of fictitious halitosis.

Suggested Reading

Bishop ER. Monosymptomatic hypochondriasis. Psychosomatics 1980; 21:731–741.

Bogdasarian RS. Halitosis. Otolaryngol Clin North Am 1986; 19:111–117.

Doty RL. Influence of age and age-related diseases on olfactory function. Ann NY Acad Sci 1989; 561:76–86.

Estrem SA, Renner G. Disorders of smell and taste. Otolaryngol Clin North Am 1987; 20:133–147.

Feldman JI, Wright HN, Leopold DA. The initial evaluation of dysosmia. Am J Otolaryngol 1986; 7:431–444.

Gent JF, Goodspeed RB, Zagrinski RT, Catalotto FA. Taste and smell problems: Validation of questions for the clinical history. Yale J Biol Med 1987; 60:27–35.

Glass BJ, Kuhel RF, Langlais RP. Treatment of common orofacial conditions. Dent Clin North Am 186; 30:421–446.

Goldberg RL, Buogiorno PA, Henkin RI. Delusions of halitosis. Psychosomatics 1985; 26:325–327, 331.

Haubrich WS. Other symptoms encountered in gastroenterologic practice. In: Berk JE, Haubrich WS, Kalser MH, Roth JLA, Schaffner F, eds. Bockus Gastroenterology. 4th ed. Philadelphia: WB Saunders, 1985:191–200.

Hawkins C. Real and imaginary halitosis. [Editorial.] Br Med J 1987; 294:200–201.

Hill DP, Jafek BW. Initial otolaryngologic assessment of patients with taste and smell disorders. Ear Nose Throat J 1989; 68:362–370.

Lamey PJ, Lewis MA. Burning mouth syndrome. Dent Update 1986; 13:185.

Powell FC. Glossodynia and other disorders of the tongue. Dermatol Clin 1987; 5:687–693.

Schiffman SS. Taste and smell disease. N Engl J Med 1983; 308:1275–1279, 1337–1343.

Scott AE. Clinical characteristics of taste and smell disorders. Ear Nose Throat J 1989; 68:297, 386.

Smith DV. Assessment of patients with taste and smell disorders. Acta Otolaryngol [Suppl] (Stockh) 1988; 458:129–133.

Tonzetich J. Direct gas-chromatographic analysis of sulfur compounds in mouth air. Arch Oral Biol 1971; 16:587–597.

INDEX

Numbers with an *f* indicate figures; numbers with a *t* indicate tables.